Radiation Therapy and the Cancer Center

Frontiers of
Radiation Therapy and
Oncology

Volume 8

Editor
JEROME M. VAETH, San Francisco, Calif.

Associate Editors
JEROLD P. GREEN, ALAN F. SCHROEDER,
SIMEON T. CANTRIL and MARY LOUISE MEURK

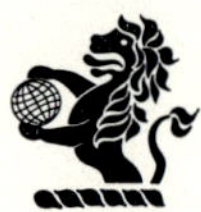

University Park Press · Baltimore · London · Tokyo

Radiation Therapy and the Cancer Center

Proceedings of the
Eighth Annual West Coast Cancer Symposium

45 figures, 10 tables, 1973

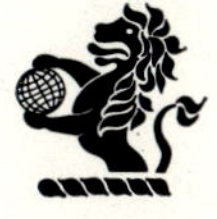

University Park Press · Baltimore · London · Tokyo

S. Karger · Basel · München · Paris · London · New York · Sydney
Arnold-Böcklin-Strasse 25, CH-4011 Basel (Switzerland)

Printed in Switzerland by Buchdruckerei Schüler AG, Biel
ISBN 3–8055–1619–3

Distributed exclusively in the United States of America and Canada by
University Park Press, Baltimore, Maryland
Library of Congress Catalog Card Number 73–11557
ISBN 0–8391–0558–4

Contents

Foreword

The eight symposium produced by the West Coast Cancer Foundation staff was entitled, Radiation Therapy and the Cancer Center. Radiation therapy or radiation oncology is the keystone of the multidiscipline center, today and the future. The specialty rightfully inherited its position based on past proven experience in Europe, Canada and the United States. Radiation therapists and their programs provide the liaison between multiple cancer specialists working in concert in clinical care, training and research for the ultimate benefit of the cancer patient. These concepts and relationships were explored in depth in San Francisco, September 22, 23, 1972.

JEROME M. VAETH, M. D.
Director
West Coast Cancer Foundation

Acknowledgement

Major support for the symposium was provided by the San Francisco Unit and the California Division of the American Cancer Society. Additional assistance was supplied by the Applied Radiation Corporation and Varian Associates.

Front. Radiation Ther. Onc., vol. 8, pp. 1–4
(Karger, Basel and University Park Press, Baltimore 1973)

Position of Multidiscipline Concept

Government Concept

B. SCHMIDT

President's Cancer Panel, New York, N. Y.

It is a great pleasure for me to be in San Francisco this morning and to open this Annual West Coast Cancer Symposium.

Since Dr. PALMER SAUNDERS from the National Cancer Institute is here to talk about the national planning in the field of cancer, and later in the day to discuss the National Cancer Institute Centers Program, I will steer largely clear of those subjects and give you a brief sketch of the background of the National Cancer Act of 1971 and the progress under that act.

I am sure that it is gratifying to those of you who are devoting your lives very largely to the cancer problem to observe that during the past 3 years, America has come of age so far as cancer research is concerned and is stepping up to its responsibilities in this respect in a way that it has never done in the past. As late as spring 1970, cancer research, like all biomedical research was on the back burner. This was true in spite of the fact that cancer was then, as it is today, the number one health concern of the American people.

A poll conducted in 1966 showed that 62% of the public feared cancer more than any other disease. Yet, of the more than 200,000,000 Americans alive today, 50,000,000 will develop cancer at present rates of incidence and 34,000,000 will die of this painful and often ugly disease if better methods of prevention and treatment are not discovered. About one-half of those deaths will occur before the age of 65, and cancer causes more deaths among children than any other disease. I do not need to point out to this audience that cancer often strikes as harshly at human dignity as at human life, and more often than not it represents financial catastrophe for the family at which it strikes.

Notwithstanding the seriousness of these figures and the depth of public concern, the amount we were spending on cancer research in 1969 was grossly inadequate. For every man, woman and child in the United State we spent in 1969: $410 on national defense; $125 on the war in Viet Nam; $19 on the space program; $19 on foreign aid; and only $0.89 on cancer research.

It was in this climate that, in the spring of 1970, Senator RALPH YARBOROUGH and the members of the Senate Committee on Labor and Public Welfare named a national panel of consultants on cancer made up of 13 distinguished scientists and doctors in the field of cancer, and 13 laymen. I had the pleasure of serving as chairman of this panel and I have never seen any group work with greater dedication and effectiveness than the professional members of our group.

The panel was charged with reporting to the Senate as promptly as possible on:

1. Where we stand today in the field of cancer;

2. What are the areas of greatest promise for significant advance; and

3. What steps should be taken to make the conquest of cancer a major national goal.

On December 4, 1970, we made our report to the Senate, setting forth the answers to these questions, and recommending specific legislation for a new and accelerated cancer initiative. A bill was promptly introduced in the Congress embodying the panel recommendations.

In January of 1971, President NIXON, in his State of the Union Address, supported the initiative recommended by the panel in these words:

'The time has come in America when the same kind of concentrated effort that split the atom and took man to the moon should be turned toward conquering this dread disease. Let us make a total national commitment to achieve this goal.'

The initial legislation implementing the recommendations of the panel was introduced in the Senate by Senator RALPH YARBOROUGH, chairman of the health subcommittee in the Senate. However, Senator YARBOROUGH did not have the opportunity of continuing his support in the Senate because he was defeated for re-election in the 1970 campaign. Senator EDWARD KENNEDY succeeded Senator YARBOROUGH as chairman of the Senate health subcommittee and he reintroduced the legislation in the new Congress in January of 1971. Cancer legislation was also introduced in the House, the most significant bill being that sponsored by Congressman PAUL ROGERS, chairman of the health subcommittee.

The proposed legislation soon became the focal points of great controversy within the scientific and medical community. It was argued that an enlarged cancer program would be at the expense of other biomedical research and medical education. None of us wanted that, but it always seemed to me that this argument was invalid because it has always been true, even from a purely selfish standpoint, that the next best thing to getting a raise yourself is for the man next door to get one. I had no doubt that increased support for cancer would promptly lead to increased support for other areas of biomedical science, and that is proving to be the case as evidenced by the recent bill, largely patterned on the cancer bill, giving substantially increased support for work in heart disease, stroke and related arterial diseases.

Other arguments against the special cancer initiative as recommended by the panel were that it would fragment biomedical research, reduce the independence of the basic researcher, attempt to program that which was not susceptible to programming, and jeopardize the system of peer review which has become widely accepted and respected in the biomedical community.

All of these matters had been most seriously considered by the panel, and it was our opinion that none of them was in fact threatened by the proposed legislation. The real basis of the conflict was a simple but important organizational issue: to what extent was the cancer effort to be independent and to what extent was it to be controlled by the director of the National Institute of Health (NIH) and to remain subject to the bureaucracy of HEW? This is the kind of issue on which the bureaucrats fight hard and supporters on both sides were rallied to the cause.

This conflict seemed to threaten the entire program for a time, but the statesmanship of the politicians resulted in the resolution of the conflict, and this was the most impressive aspect of the entire experience so far as I was concerned. President NIXON supported the panel, and his leadership was invaluable. Senator KENNEDY made it clear that his only interest was in getting the best possible cancer bill and that he would do anything helpful to that end, including the withdrawal of his bill in favor of the Administration bill, thus foregoing what might have been thought to be his personal political advantage. In the House of Representatives, the dynamic leadership, the industry and the dedication of the health subcommittee chairman, Congressman PAUL ROGERS, and the ingenuity and wisdon of the ranking minority member, ANCHER NELSEN, also greatly facilitated the ultimate legislation.

Thus, we had a situation where President NIXON, Senator EDWARD KENNEDY, Senator JAVITS, Senator DOMINICK, Congressman ROGERS, Congressman NELSEN, and many, many others of all shades of political persuasion worked together in harmony to produce the Cancer Act of 1971. This was a very impressive display of unity in subordinating partisan and personal interest to the public good. I believe that this act gives us the foundation we need on which to build the best cancer research program of which American medicine and American science is capable.

The act was signed into law on December 23, 1971, but the impact of the new cancer initiative was already being seen in the funding of the national cancer program. In the fiscal year ending June 30, 1970, $181,000,000 was appropriated for cancer. In 1971, the figure rose to $227,500,000, in 1972, we had $378,000,000 and for the current year, I anticipate an appropriation in the neighborhood of $490,000,000. There were $492,000,000 in the HEW bill that was vetoted, but I have been personally assured by the President that this veto was in no part aimed at the cancer funds.

No one is under any illusion that simply spending more money will solve the cancer problem. There was much more behind the timing of the new cancer initiative than that. There is no question in my mind that we have today more opportunities in cancer research and more promising areas for accelerated exploration than have ever heretofore existed. In the fields of cell biology, cell surface phenomena, molecular biology, immunology, virology, etiology and early diagnosis, as well as chemotherapy, radiation therapy and surgery, we have new insights which in my judgment can lead to far better methods of prevention, detection and control of cancer than have heretofore been available. It was for these reasons that an enhanced and accelerated program was advocated at this time.

Cancer is an implacable foe. It is many diseases, not one, and it will probably not lend itself to a single form of immunization or a single cure. However, I am convinced that we can make far more rapid progress against cancer under the new program, and we owe it to the people of our nation and of the world to do so. Without raising false hopes and without creating false optimism, we must give to the American people the best program in cancer research and cancer control of which American medicine and American science is capable. Such a program must do two things: Firstly, we must do everything possible through research to expand our knowledge as rapidly and as intelligently as possible. Secondly, we must, meanwhile, do everything within our power to see that our present knowledge is applied as early as possible in the most effective way to prevent or control cancer among our people today.

I know that most of you are dedicating your lives to that and, for that, I salute you.

Thank you again for your generosity and for the opportunity to join you in your meeting here this morning. I wish you a most successful meeting.

Author's address: Mr. B. SCHMIDT, 630 Fifth Avenue, *New York, N Y 10020* (USA)

Front. Radiation Ther. Onc., vol. 8, pp. 5–17
(Karger, Basel and University Park Press, Baltimore 1973)

Development of the National Cancer Program Plan

J. P. SAUNDERS

Division of Cancer Grants, National Cancer Institute, Bethesda, Md.

New Cancer Initiative

In 1971 President NIXON, in his State of the Union Speech and Health Message, called for an intensified attack on cancer and stated that he was asking the Congress for additional funds for expanded research and development efforts. He called for commitments to a national program for the conquest of cancer. The Congress initiated such a program by providing an increased regular appropriation and additional supplementary funds for the National Cancer Institute. On December 23, 1971, President NIXON signed into law the National Cancer Act of 1971, culminating a year-long effort to launch an unprecedented attack on cancer.

The importance of a national plan was stressed by the panel of consultants established by the Senate in 1970 to review the cancer field and make recommendations for an expanded effort in cancer. Administration testimony also indicated the need for an overall plan. Toward this end, the National Cancer Institute formulated a plan outline and called upon the scientific community to participate in the full development of the National Cancer Program Plan.

In addition to discussions with the National Advisory Cancer Council, the American Association of Cancer Institutes, and others, 250 prominent scientists and physician investigators, representing a broad spectrum of biomedical and clinical disciplines,[1] met in a series of 41 planning sessions

---

1 Suggestions for participants were invited from the American Association for Cancer Research, The American Association for the Advancement of Science, the American Cancer Society, the American Society of Therapeutic Radiologists, the American Surgical Association, each of the Federated Societies for Experimental Biology, the National Academy of Sciences, the Society of University Surgeons, the participants themselves, and the NCI staff.

and 2 major review sessions held between October 1971 and March 1972 for the purpose of developing a scientific and operational foundation for a National Cancer Program.

Purpose, Scope and Content of the NCPP

The Congressional Committee[2] report on the National Cancer Attack Act of 1971 stated that the plan should initially cover a 5 year period and that 'each year the Director shall prepare a program plan for the next five years. The requirement would provide the Nation with a continuously updated national plan'. It was felt that this 'rolling plan' mechanism would allow the National Cancer Institute, the President and the Congress to take advantage of new opportunities as they arise.

The National Cancer Program Plan (NCPP) is to be the vehicle for coordinating, monitoring and reporting progress of the National Cancer Program. It will be the primary basis for the cancer research dialogue between the scientific community and the President, Congress and the public (fig. 1). The NCPP will make it possible to:

1. Focus and relate the necessary multidisciplinary scientific approaches to objectives couched in appropriate language so they can be generally evaluated and understood by the public.

2. Provide the basic and scientific and managerial guidelines for program decisions and actions resulting from advances in scientific knowledge and changes in resource constraints.

The NCPP will be an integrated, operational plan for conducting a systematic attack on the problems of cancer. The more important aspects of the plan are:

1. It will be an implementable plan which represents scientific courses of action that can be actively pursued, or immediately implemented, when the plan is approved and required resources are provided.

2. It will be an integrated plan to encompass current federal and non-federal cancer research programs and additional courses of action permissible under an expanded, intensified effort.

2   House of Representatives Subcommittee on Public Health and Environment of the Committee on Interstate and Foreign Commerce.

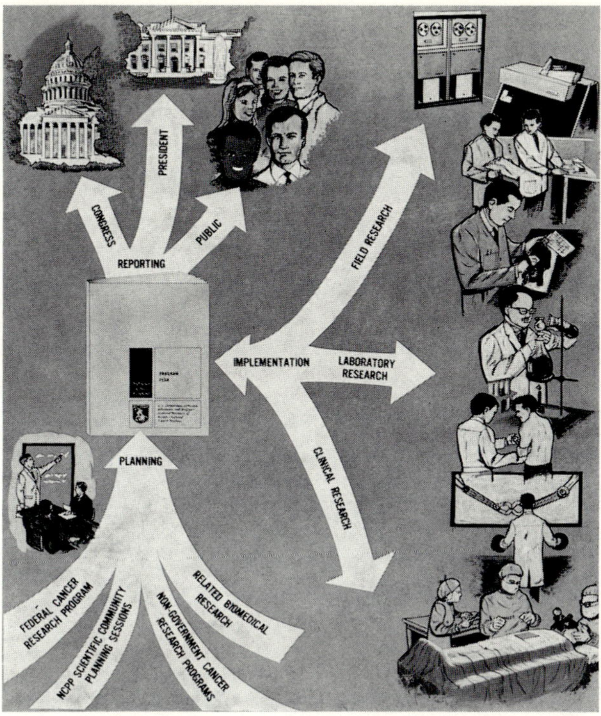

Fig. 1. Planning-Implementation-Reporting Interactions of the National Cancer Program Plan.

3. It will be comprehensive in scope since it will include scientific efforts directed toward all facets of the cancer problem (cause and prevention, detection and diagnosis, therapy and rehabilitation) and conducted over the entire research spectrum (basic, applied and developmental).

National Cancer Program Strategy

The overall National Cancer Program Strategy consists of two inter-related strategy components and associated hierarchies (fig. 2):

1. Research strategy – delineates the scientific courses of actions to achieve the program objectives and goal.

2. Operational strategy – delineates the management courses of action to implement the research strategy.

NATIONAL PROGRAM STRATEGY
COMPONENTS

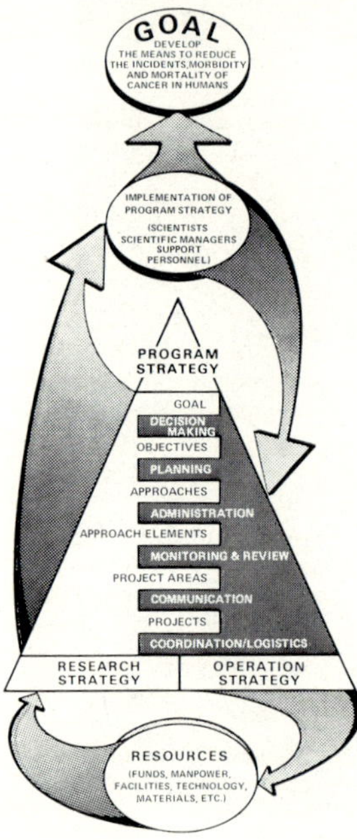

Fig. 2. National program strategy components.

There is an important conceptual difference between research and operational strategies. The recognition of this difference has a direct impact on the philosophy and character of program management.

The sole purpose of the research strategy is to provide the logical organization of the scientific research and development required to accomplish the program goal (key cancer objectives, approaches, approach elements, project areas and projects). The current state of scientific knowledge is the only basis for the formulation of the research strategy. As the state of knowledge in various areas of the research strategy advances, the content and organization of the strategy may change. However, it remains independent from such considerations as resource constraints, mechanisms of support, review procedures, etc., which have no impact on the scientific content of the research strategy. The scientific community will participate in the updating of the research strategy through planning sessions similar to those held for the initial formulation of the NCPP.

The operational strategy represents the organization of the key program managerial functions (planning, decision-making, administration, review and monitoring, coordination, communication and resources, development and allocation) (fig. 2). Its only purpose is to provide an optimal basis for effective, efficient and timely translation of the research strategy into those actions which have a high probability of achieving the cancer objectives with the most productive use of required resources (which are always limited in the totality). It, too, must change as research requirements change and as more productive organizational and operational patterns are developed. However, it remains dependent upon the research strategy for its purpose, which is to be responsive and supportive to the needs of research.

Although the research and operational strategies are discussed separately, it is the continuous blending of these two elements into an operating system that is critical to the success of the program. The strategy elements in combination provide a reference baseline for conducting the program by:

1. Facilitating decision-making at all levels.

2. Providing maximum visibility of program activities.

3. Permitting the rapid and efficient incorporation of new ideas, leads, etc., in all levels of the program.

4. Facilitating redirection when opportunities and unforeseen problems occur.

The blending of the two strategy components is not an easy task and cannot be accomplished by any one group of people. The National Cancer Program can be achieved only through the effective interlinking of the efforts of the President, the President's Cancer Panel, the National Cancer Advisory Board, the National Cancer Institute director and staff, and the working scientists who will constitute the operating core of the program. The NCPP will provide the basis for a common dialogue and, thus, greatly facilitate this critical interlinking which will result in a cohesive and coordinated national effort in cancer.

The National Cancer Program research strategy is the combination of selected laboratory, field and clinical research courses of action necessary to achieve the program objectives and goal. To facilitate planning and implementation of the program research strategy, it has been organized in a hierarchical format with the following levels (fig. 2): (1) national program goal; (2) national program objective; (3) approaches; (4) approach elements, and (5) project areas.

The hierarchical structure provides continuing focus on constant, disease-oriented objectives. The research strategy structure and organization is dynamic and facilitates the inclusion of new research to achieve the objectives at all levels of the hierarchy.

National Cancer Program Goal

As we have seen, the program goal is the first or top level in the research strategy hierarchy. The ultimate cancer research goal is the 'Development of means for the prevention of all cancers in man' (fig. 3). This goal is too general and long-term to provide a basis for formulating a specific research program and measuring progress. Therefore, the National Cancer Program goal has been defined as the 'Development of means for the significant reduction of the incidence, morbidity and mortality of cancer in man'. In this way the National Cancer Program goal achievement can be assessed in terms, for instance, of improvement in the percentages of successes for each

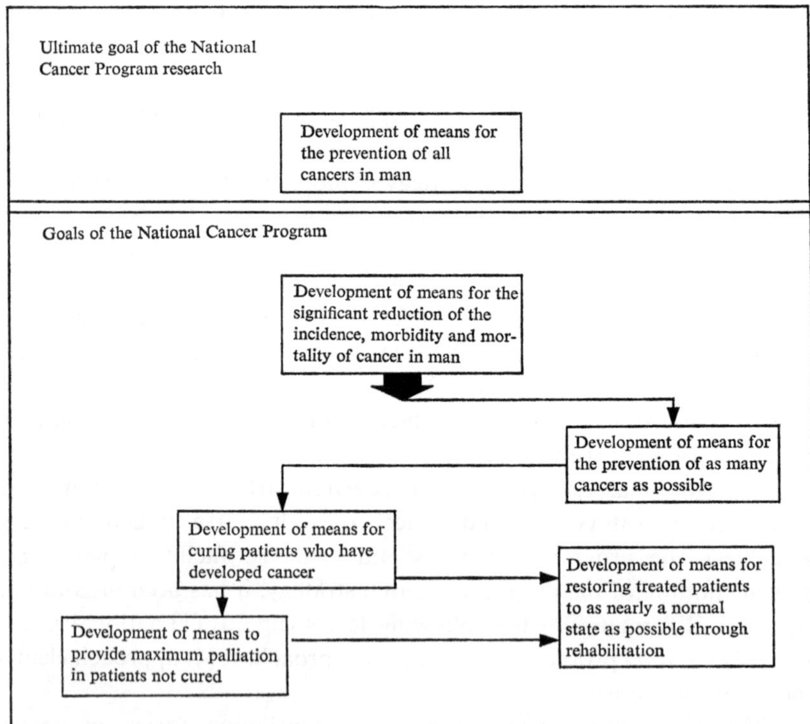

Fig. 3. Goal of the National Cancer Program.

stage of cancer, i.e. cause and prevention, detection and diagnosis, therapy and rehabilitation. The major thrusts to achieve the goal include: (1) prevention; (2) treatment (curing), and (3) palliation and rehabilitation.

National Cancer Program Objectives

The second level of the research hierarchy consists of the key cancer program objectives (fig. 4). These objectives are based on a conceptual scheme of cancer as a process which can be attacked by:

1. Preventing as many cancers as possible.

2. Curing (through detection, diagnosis and treatment) as many cancers as possible.

3. Rehabilitating and palliating those patients cured and those not cured.

The objectives are defined this way because:

1. They encompass all aspects of cancer research – research on the nature, cause, prevention, detection, diagnosis and prognosis, therapy and rehabilitation.

2. They are related directly to the National Cancer Program goal, since their achievement will contribute to the achievement of that goal.

3. They are stated in lay-oriented terminology for reporting National Cancer Program progress to the President, the Congress and the public.

*National Cancer Program Approaches, Approach Elements
and Project Areas*

The remaining levels of the research hierarchy include the: (1) approaches; (2) approach elements, and (3) project areas.

An approach is a broad plan of attack which singly or in combination with other related approaches forms the basis for research programs to achieve a particular National Cancer Program objective. An approach is a major research thrust based on multidisciplinary research efforts and consists of approach elements, project areas and projects.

The approach elements are major components of an approach which in combination (or possibly singly) with related approach elements will contribute to the successful implementation of the approach. Each approach element has its own objective which can be monitored and evaluated in terms of progress toward supporting the approach in the achievement of its program objective.

Each project area is an aggregate of individual research projects which collectively and in combination with related project areas support the achievement of the approach element to which it belongs. Each project area

Research phase	Key cancer program objectives
Prevention	1. Develop the means to reduce the effectiveness of external agents in increasing the probabilities of development of cancers in existing individuals or subsequent generations
	2. Develop the means to modify individuals (e. g., by vaccination) to decrease the likelihood of cancer development, both in the current generation and in subsequent offspring
	3. Develop the means to prevent conversions of cells to those capable of forming cancers (i. e., block, or interfere with the proximate step, or steps, involved in conversion to cells capable of forming cancers)
	4. Develop the means to prevent tumor establishment from cells already capable of forming cancers (e. g., transformed cells, cells constituting precancerous tissues, and cells from primary tumors that lodge elsewhere in the body in a metastatic state, either active or dormant)
Detection, Diagnosis, Prognosis	5. Develop the means to achieve an accurate assessment of the presence, extent and probable course of cancer risks in population groups (including attention to precancerous lesions) and of cancers in individuals alone (diagnosis) and in groups (detection) as an aid to prevention, cure or prognosis
Therapy	6. Develop the means to cure as many patients as possible and to maintain maximum control of the cancerous process in patients not cured
Rehabilitation	7. Develop the means to restore patients with residual defects as a consequence of their disease or treatment to as nearly a normal functioning state as possible

Fig. 4. National Cancer Program objectives.

has its own objective which can be monitored and evaluated in terms of progress toward supporting the approach element in the achievement of its objective.

Organization of the NCPP Development

The development of the NCPP has been organized into 6 phases:
Phase I   – formulation of NCPP framework.
Phase II   – approaches planning sessions.
Phase III – project areas planning sessions.
Phase IV – analysis and integration of inputs.
Phase V   – preparation of the strategic plan.
Phase VI – preparation of the operational plan.
41 planning sessions were held between October 1971 and January 1972 at Airlie House, Warrenton, Virginia. These sessions were divided into groups: (1) the *approaches* planning sessions, and (2) the *project area* planning sessions.

Approaches Planning Sessions

The approaches planning sessions were directed toward developing broad plans of attack for achieving the 7 key cancer objectives (fig. 5). These sessions, which involved 39 scientists organized into 7 panels (one for each objective), provided recommendations for both the research and operational strategies. The research strategy recommendations were presented in the form of 36 specific scientific approaches and associated approach elements deemed to be the minimum number of major research thrusts judged necessary to achieve the key cancer program objectives. The operational strategy recommendations were general guidance on the organization and management structure for implementing the overall strategic plan. The outputs of these sessions are covered in 7 separate reports.

Project Area Planning Sessions

The project area planning sessions were directed toward developing more detailed descriptions of the research necessary to carry out the ap-

Overall program strategy

Research strategy		Operational strategy	
Purpose	Outputs	Purpose	Outputs
Provide a logical conceptual unconstrained, scientific framework for the overall strategic plan	*Approaches –* miminum number of major research thrusts judged necessary to achieve the key cancer program objective *Approach elements –* description of the major research components of the approach	Provide general guidance on the organization and management structure for implementing the overall strategic plan	Describe general guidance concerning: organization management

Fig. 5. Approaches session, purpose and guidance.

Overall program strategy

Research strategy		Operational strategy	
Purpose	Outputs	Purpose	Outputs
Provide a scientifically sound research base for the major research thrusts	Descriptions of the minimum number of *project areas* necessary to implement the approaches Descriptions of the *project areas* in terms of a set of laboratory field and clinical research projects	Provide guidance on the resources required to accomplish the various research components	Describe resources necessary to implement the project area in terms of: money manpower technology facilities equipment information materials

Fig. 6. Project area planning sessions, purpose and guidance.

proaches developed in the approaches planning sessions (fig. 6). These project area planning sessions, which involved 211 scientists organized into 34 panels (one panel per approach)[3] also provided recommendations for both the research and operational strategies. The research recommendations were presented in the form of 150 approach elements and 764 project areas deemed to be the minimum number required to implement the initial approaches. The project areas recommended by the planning sessions defined the research objective, key research events, present status, time-frame, progress criteria, impact, probability of success and relative priority (fig. 7). The operational strategy recommendations were estimates of the resources (money, manpower, facilities, etc.) necessary to implement the project areas recommended. The outputs of these sessions are covered in 33 separate reports.

(a) Project area objective	What is the major problem to be solved?
(b) Project area description	How will we solve it?
(c) Key research events	What is critical to success of the project area?
(d) Present research status	Where are we now?
(e) Research inputs required	Where are the prerequisites for this project?
(f) Form of results	Reports, vaccines, equipment, models, etc.
(g) Research time frame	Short-term: less than 5 years Long-term: 5 years or longer
(h) Progress criteria	Scientific milestones
(i) Impact on approach element of successful achievement of objective	High Medium Low Include 3 criteria of impact in order of importance
(j) Probability of successful achievement of objective	High Medium Low Include 3 criteria for probability of success in order of importance
(k) Relative priority of project area	High Medium Low Include up to 3 criteria for priority selection in order of importance

Fig. 7. Project area level of definition.

3   Objective 7 (rehabilitation) approaches were detailed in the approaches session.

Status of the NCPP

In addition to the planning sessions, Dr. CARL G. BAKER, then the director of the National Cancer Institute, through a letter published in the journal *Science,* invited members of the scientific community to submit ideas for consideration in the national plan. All of this material is being used to formulate the initial overall plan for the National Cancer Program. The documentation for the NCPP will consist of 3 volumes (fig. 8).

The NCPP is an hierarchy of plans composed of a strategic plan, operational plan and specific individual scientific program plans. The plans within this hierarchy vary in detail. Each succeeding level is more detailed than the previous one. The strategic plan presents the major national objectives, major courses of actions and estimated resources necessary to achieve the objectives. This plan presents the basic framework and direction for the overall program. The operational plan will include more detailed information concerning specific program milestones, scientific subobjectives and plans for implementation. This plan will provide the detail necessary to monitor and control the national program. The individual scientific program plans (e.g., chemotherapy, special virus cancer program, cancer control program and the organ site programs) will include the detail necessary for day-to-day program operations, monitoring and reporting.

Volume I. The Executive Summary
A brief presentation of the main features of the strategic plan, including research and operational strategies and the preliminary 1974-1978 resources plan

Volume II. The Strategic Plan
Part 1. Research and Operational Strategies
A full accounting of the organization and development of the strategic plan including descriptions of the components of the research and operational strategies and the 1974-1978 resources plan

Part 2. Digest of Scientific Research Recommendations
A digest of over 3,000 pages of material developed during the 41 planning sessions arranged according to the 7 key cancer objectives

Volume III. The Program Operating Plan
This volume is currently under development and is scheduled for completion during 1973. It will delineate the program milestones and subjectives necessary to monitor and control the national program

---

Fig. 8. Documentation for the National Cancer Program Plan.

Because of the importance of this plan, it is undergoing extensive, in-depth review by the National Academy of Sciences, Office of Science and Technology, Office of Management and Budget, Secretary DHEW, Director NIH (including his staff and advisory committee), Presidential Cancer Panel, National Cancer Advisory Board, planning session participants and the National Cancer Institute senior staff.

The apparent extension of time of the submission of the strategic plan has in no way delayed the implementation of the plan. The current research program is now reflecting the implementation of many of the concepts developed during the planning effort.

The strategic and operational plans will in no way constrain the science investigations needed to achieve the program goal. The plans will undergo constant revision to reflect the latest findings, leads and opportunities. As with the development of the initial plan, the scientific community will continue to be involved in the program planning. It will only be through the continued collective effort of all persons involved in cancer research and control that the conquest of cancer will be achieved.

Author's address: Dr. J. PALMER SAUNDERS, Director, Division of Cancer Grants, National Cancer Institute, *Bethesda, MD 20014* (USA)

Front. Radiation Ther. Onc., vol. 8, pp. 18–25
(Karger, Basel and University Park Press, Baltimore 1973)

Radiation Therapy and the Cancer Center

The Rôle of the American Cancer Society

J. J. STEIN

UCLA Center for Health Saences, Los Angeles, Calif.

To the layman, the term 'cancer center' means a center from which he can expect to get the latest information concerning cancer, and the best treatment available. ADAMS [1], although a layman, has described the cancer center as many of us who are physicians devoting our major professional interest to cancer would like to think of it – 'The cancer center appears to be the ideal combination of the features essential to cancer research: the collaboration between the clinician and the research scientist; the collaboration of the many biomedical disciplines; the availability of the latest technologic developments, and the opportunity to concentrate on targeted clinical problems and to solve them through teamed basic and clinical research.'

A tremendous impetus has been given toward a successful approach to this goal by the recently enacted legislation which provides means for a comprehensive program for the conquest of the cancer problem. This program must include studies aimed at the prevention of cancer, e.g. lung cancer, for the continued investigation of the rôle of viruses, endogenous and exogenous factors, of molecular, biological, biochemical, hormonal and immunological influences, and of new chemotherapeutic agents.

The education of physicians in the latest treatment methods and diagnostic procedures must be kept ahead of the general enlightenment of the population. Success or failure in the treatment of patients with cancer too often may depend on the knowledge and competence of the first physician the patient consults. If the patient is not given the proper advice or treatment, he may not obtain an adequate result when such an outcome could be successful.

Existing cancer centers and medical and research centers with a special interest in cancer have demonstrated their importance by providing leadership plus collaborative efforts between the basic scientist and the clinician. Treatment techniques have been improved because of having adequate numbers of patients with different types of cancer, staff with expertise and motivation, and excellent research and clinical equipment.

Two very important features of the cancer center are the provision of an intellectual environment, and communications. The close proximity of the scientists engaged in basic research with the clinicians, and the awareness of each of the others' problems is most helpful. If really adequate communications existed today between the professions and the laity, two of every three patients with cancer could be cured instead of one of every three so afflicted, utilizing present-day diagnostic and therapeutic methods.

Even with the strengthening of existing cancer centers and the establishment of 15 new large cancer centers strategically located about the country, there should be no cause for alarm or fear from existing medical centers or from the medical profession.

The existing specialized cancer hospitals and institutes and research centers have contributed greatly to our present knowledge of cancer diagnosis, treatment, research and cancer prevention. They have also been actively involved in postgraduate education for physicians, scientists and paramedical personnel.

Approximately 60% of all the hospitals in the United States have 100 beds or less, and 85% of all patients with benign and malignant neoplastic disease are treated in community hospitals that are not affiliated with medical schools [7]. Patients like to be treated close to their homes and families, and rightfully so.

It can be estimated that for the United States as a whole, there will probably be about 260 to 270 new cancer cases diagnosed each year per 100,000 population (excluding carcinoma *in situ* and basal and squamous cell skin cancer). Only a small portion of the patients with cancer could actually be treated in the cancer centers. The centers would be fully engaged in the perfection of treatment techniques, study of combinations of therapy, investigations of potential cancer tests for screening purposes, the management of certain types of cancer, the use of highly sophisticated techniques, and many other basic problems [8].

Great progress has been made in the management of patients with Hodgkin's disease, the non-Hodgkin's malignant lymphomas, retinoblastomas, Wilms' tumors, and other malignant tumors where it has been possible to have enough patients, teams of specialists, adequately trained personnel and excellent equipment. The cancer center can provide excellent radiation therapy and dosimetry equipment and can attract well trained radiation therapists, physicists, dosimetrists, and provide opportunities for research.

The main functions of the cancer centers would be to provide specialized training, to develop and evaluate new techniques for diagnosis and treatment, to manage patients presenting special problems, to offer special education for the community physicians, and to cooperate closely with all voluntary, local, state and federal agencies engaged in health activities. The participation by the practicing physician is essential for the success of any cancer program.

The majority of Americans today are unaware of the new governmental program for the conquest of cancer. There is a great need for public education and public information. The American Cancer Society has many volunteers engaged in public education endeavors. Efforts are being made to recruit the estimated 200,000 additional public information volunteers needed to carry out minimum activities and to provide opportunities for their training and guidance. The society plans to have one volunteer for every 1,000 members of the population.

In a study made at the request of the society to determine the potential impact of the increased government cancer research program on the people's willingness to contribute to the American Cancer Society, it was found that about 3 of 10 people (30%) reported that they are aware that the government has recently expanded its cancer research program. One-half of this group, who believe that the government has increased its cancer research effort, believe that the research of the American Cancer Society is more important because cancer is a major problem, that a multiple effort is needed, and that there is a general need for more and continued cancer research. Very few people believed that there would be a duplication of research effort. The total data from this study indicate that the increased expenditures by the government for cancer research have not lessened the people's commitment to the American Cancer Society program [5].

The society has vast network through which it can hope eventually to reach all individuals in this country. There are, in addition to the national office with its highly competent staff, 57 divisions and 3,100 units. There are approximately 2,225,000 volunteers who are unceasingly working toward the total control of cancer and 'to eventually put themselves out of business when this is accomplished'.

The medical and lay volunteers and the staff of the society have worked tirelessly for many years in order that the attack on cancer would become a national goal and be recognized as such by the federal government. In 1971, with the passing of the National Cancer Act by the Congress and the signing of the act by President NIXON, the conquest of cancer received a tremendous boost.

Since 1948, about $300,000,000 has been awarded by the American Cancer Society for research. In 1971, more than $25,000,000 was allocated for cancer research by the society and its divisions [10].

The society was helpful in getting legislation passed which established the National Cancer Institute in 1937. This legislation also created the National Advisory Cancer Council.

The society has been continuously working since its inception to get anyone and everyone; the federal government, the state governments and their subdivisions, and the general public, all working for the successful control of cancer.

The society repeatedly testified before congressional groups emphasizing the need for concerted action against cancer. Most certainly, it was at least partially a result of these efforts that the senate appointed a National Panel of Consultants on the Conquest of Cancer. Six of the consultants were members of the board of directors of the society.

President NIXON sent a letter dated November 2, 1971, which was read at the Annual 1971 Dinner Meeting of the society. The following paragraph is quoted from the letter: 'In making a commitment to the conquest of cancer, this nation is undertaking one of its greatest endeavors. This commitment is immeasurably strengthened by being a total one – representing the combined efforts of Government and citizen resources and bolstered by the dedication of the volunteer workers against cancer who are organized under the symbol of the "Sword of Hope", the American Cancer Society' [3].

Since the title of this symposium is 'Radiation Therapy and the Cancer Center', it should be noted that one of the major provisions of the new National Cancer Act is to authorize the director of the National Cancer Institute 'to provide for the establishment of fifteen new centers for clinical research, training, and demonstration of advanced diagnostic and treatment methods relating to cancer' [4].

In the same section (section 408) of the National Cancer Act of 1971, the following statement is made: 'Section 408 (b) The Director of the National Cancer Institute, under policies established by the Director of the National Institutes of Health and after consultation with the National Cancer Advisory Board, is authorized to enter into cooperative agreements with public or private non-profit agencies or institutions to pay all or part of the cost of planning, establishing, or strengthening, and providing basic operating support for existing or new centers including, but not limited to, centers established under subsection (a) for clinical research, training, and demonstration of advanced diagnostic and treatment methods relating to cancer.' Subsection (a) relates to the establishment of 15 new centers [4].

There must be a real attempt at wide geographic distribution of the new centers, for the whole objective is to improve the management of patients with cancer at all levels, but in particular at the community level.

It is hoped that great care will go into developing and planning the cancer centers so that they will be located on the basis of need, that they will really be wanted by the medical community, and will be used by the entire community. It is further hoped that grants will not be allocated to those who see this merely as an opportunity to get funds, but who have no real knowledge of the goals for the conquest of cancer and of the research, education, and services required for the total management of patients with cancer.

The patient with curable cancer will have his best opportunity to obtain a good result when radiation therapy centers which are well equipped, and staffed with adequate personnel both in the clinical and investigative fields, are established.

The first physician who sees the patient with cancer and who undertakes or recommends the method of therapy to be used will largely determine whether a successful result will be obtained. Of malignant tumors which are potentially curable, for 50% of the patients surgery will be the treatment of choice, and for about 40%, radiation therapy used singly or in combination with other treatment methods will be preferred.

Real progress will be made when more radiation therapy treatment centers are established and when the training of radiation therapists is separated from diagnostic radiology.

STEIN [9], in 1967, made the following comment: 'The trend in radiation therapy is for the separation of radiation therapy or therapeutic radiology from diagnostic radiology, towards the use of megavolt X-rays and electrons; greater understanding of radiobiology and radiation physics; the centralization of equipment and establishment of radiation therapy centers; the use of combined modalities (e.g., preoperative radiation therapy combined with surgery, and of radiation therapy combined with chemotherapy and surgery); and to challenge preconceived "statements of fact" as dogma.'

DEL REGATO [2] stated that in 1939 there were only 49 physicians in the United States who were practicing radiation therapy exclusively. Also, that in 1960 there were only 25 residents in training in 'straight' radiation therapy in the United States, in 1970, 180, and in 1972 there were 256 residents in 'straight' radiation therapy. There were 452 active American members of the American Society of Therapeutic Radiologists in 1972. There is a great need for many more well trained radiation therapists.

The government cannot accomplish the conquest of cancer alone. At the time of the signing of the National Cancer Act, the following statement was made by President NIXON: 'In saying there will be a Presidential commitment, a Congressional commitment, and a government commitment, I should emphasize that a total national commitment means more than government. It means all the voluntary activities must continue... The new National cancer program must not replace our present efforts to fight cancer, it must supplement and build on them... It is essential that an organization such as the American Cancer Society which has done so much to promote research and education in this field, continue to play its effective role' [10].

Even though the government intends to spend large sums of money for the conquest of cancer, the American Cancer Society intends to increase its own efforts in research, education, and service, for there will be greater need than ever for all of its services.

The Society maintains a great deal of flexibility and it can in a short period of time change its directions or institute and fund new programs wherever needed.

There will be a continuing demand for funds for basic and clinical research. The society has never had adequate funds to support all meritorious project requests. The society may permit great freedom of action in research and greater flexibility. Also, if the funds are granted for a certain period, they are not later reduced or cancelled. The Research Professorship Program of this society was begun in 1957. There are 22 highly qualified scientists who have lifetime American Cancer Society Professorships in centers of research in this country.

With the establishment of new cancer centers and the strengthening of others, there will be a greater need than ever for professional education for physicians, dentists, medical and dental students and nurses.

The society awards clinical fellowships to physicians and dentists to further their knowledge in the diagnosis and treatment of cancer and also advanced fellowships for junior faculty members who have completed their formal training for eligibility for the American Board Certification in their specialty.

Over 30 teaching films have been produced. An excellent clinical journal for physicians called CA is distributed to over 300,000 individuals every 2 months. An outstanding journal called *Cancer* is published monthly under the aegis of the society.

National conferences on cancer of the colon and rectum and breast have been well attended. Additional conferences on these subjects have been held or will be held, as well as national conferences on genitourinary cancer and cancer nursing. National conferences on cancer are held every 4 years and are cosponsored with the National Cancer Institute. A research and clinical conference on staging in Hodgkin's disease has been sponsored by the society.

The Program of Professorships of Clinical Oncology of the society was established in 1971 to 'bring about more effective management of cancer patients by improving cancer teaching in medical schools and other approlpriate institutions at undergraduate, graduate, and continuing education levels, and to extend the benefits of such teaching to both students and practitioners of the medical, dental, nursing and allied health professions', and to 'foster cooperation of all relevant medical and scientific disciplines in the management of cancer' [6].

Task forces have been planned and approved by the society to conquer uterine cancer, for the control of breast cancer, and for the study of possible occupational and nonoccupational carcinogenic agents with the cooperation of labor and industry.

The society occupies a unique position in that it has such a great number of dedicated volunteers, both professional and nonprofessional, who will be able to provide communications for people to people programs and to 'get the word out' as quickly as possible. Also, the physicians, dentists and nurses should learn what new developments are taking place as soon as possible after discoveries are made in the laboratories and made available to the practicing physician.

The society is delighted to see the national commitment for the conquest of cancer, and is willing to cooperate to the fullest extent with the federal governmental agencies, with state, county and all levels of government and with other voluntary organizations in an effort to eradicate cancer. There is no spirit of competition, only one of mutual assistance.

The service and rehabilitation efforts of the society have been outstanding. The services rendered to the patients who have had mastectomies, laryngectomies, ostomies and amputations has been outstanding. The major efforts for the control of cancer quackery have been made by volunteers of the society.

The American Cancer Society is the largest and most effective voluntary health organization in the world. It has done more than any one organization to focus the attention of the nation on the seriousness of cancer as a major health problem.

The society is able to render its valuable service to the professions and to the laity through the financing of research, providing professional and lay education and information, and through its service efforts. The goal of the society is to accelerate and to help coordinate all efforts in the research, clinical and service categories leading toward the eventual control of cancer.

References

1   ADAMS, L. W.: Cancer centers and the American people. Cancer, Philad. *29:* 821–823 (1972).
2   REGATO, J. A. DEL: The American Society of Therapeutic Radiologists. Cancer, Philad. *29:* 1443–1445 (1972).
3   American Cancer Society: Annual report 1971, p. 5 (American Cancer Society Inc., New York 1972).
4   The National Cancer Act of 1971. Cancer, Philad. *29:* 917–923 (1972).
5   American Cancer Society: The potential impact of the increased government cancer research program on people's willingness to contribute to the American Cancer Society (American Cancer Society Inc., New York 1972).
6   American Cancer Society: Policies governing grants for support of Professorships of Clinical Oncology (American Cancer Society Inc., New York 1971).
7   ROSS, W. L.: Personal communication (1966).
8   STEIN, J. J.: Radiation therapy and the cancer problem. Med. Times *97:* 123–128 (1969).
9   STEIN, J. J.: Trends in the management of the cancer patient. The president's address 1966. Amer. J. Roentgenol. *99:* 279–288 (1967).
10 American Cancer Society: What the new federal cancer programs means to the American Cancer Society (American Cancer Society Inc., New York 1972).

Author's adress: Dr. JUSTIN J. STEIN, Radiation Therapy Division, UCLA Center for Health Sciences, *Los Angeles, CA 90024* (USA)

Front. Radiation Ther. Onc., vol. 8, pp. 26–28
(Karger, Basel and University Park Press, Baltimore 1973)

Radiation Therapy and the Cancer Center

The Advisory Function of the Committee for Radiation Therapy Studies

S. KRAMER

Department of Radiation Therapy, Thomas Jefferson University Hospital,
Philadelphia, Pa.

I shall introduce my subject by reporting briefly on the history and function of the Committee for Radiation Therapy Studies (CRTS). This committee was initiated in 1959 through the combined efforts of the Radiation Study Section and the National Cancer Institute (NCI), to serve informally as a committee for radiation therapists to assist in the development of clinical trials in radiation therapy. Initially the committee consisted of senior radiation therapists of this country who had special expertise in those areas of radiation therapy in which clinical trials seemed likely to be of benefit. The first cooperative clinical study, on 'Preoperative radiation in lung cancer', was launched in 1961. The committee remained relatively inactive until October 1963 when, at the urging of Dr. RALPH MEADER, then Associate Director of Extramural Programs for the NCI, Dr. GILBERT FLETCHER, chairman of the original committee, was asked to reactivate the committee, to increase its membership and to expand its aims beyond the designing of clinical trials. It was agreed by both the committee members and the NCI staff that this committee would remain a group of 'private citizens', free to determine its own projects relative to its particular interests, to select its membership according to committee choice, and to define its organization as it deemed sufficient and necessary.

Dr. GILBERT FLETCHER chaired this group from its inception until the end of 1971, and under his wise guidance, and with the support of, and interaction with, the staff of the extramural program of the NCI, the committee rapidly expanded its function beyond the initiation of clinical trials (without, however, neglecting these – it launched three more cooperative studies by 1967). The committee functioned by responding to requests from the NCI for opinions and advice on research aspects of radiation therapy, on training in radiation therapy and manpower needs in radiation therapy; and it has found the NCI most responsive. Indeed, it is a matter of record that the extramural program of the NCI has done a great deal to advance and support our field in many ways.

In addition, the committee, either from discussion within itself or stimulation by members of the radiation therapy community, has dealt with questions and problems affecting our specialty and particularly so, as it interfaces with other related fields in cancer. In conjunction with the Radiation Study Section and the National Academy of Sciences, it has sponsored a number of conferences, bringing together radiobiologists and clinicians, with the 1969 Carmel Conference being perhaps the most successful of these. The CRTS also laid the groundwork and provided the initial support for the Radiologic Physics Center of the American Association of Physicists in Medicine. This physics center is now independently supported by the NCI in supervising the dosimetric and other radiologic physics aspects of a great many clinical trials involving radiation therapy.

One of the major thrusts of our committee has been an effort to define the rôle of radiation therapy in cancer management, and this, of course, has led to involvement in the cancer center program. Among the many types of cancer centers supported in the past, there has been a number of radiation therapy research centers. In advising on the multidisciplinary or comprehensive cancer centers now receiving prominence, the CRTS has taken the stand that radiation therapy, or *radiation oncology*, as it is better called, must be the keystone of a comprehensive or multidisciplinary center since radiation oncology is the one specialty totally devoted to cancer management. We have long espoused the multidisciplinary approach to the cancer patient for optimal decision-making and care; and in our clinical practice we have developed considerable expertise in collaborating with our colleagues, setting up joint clinics, etc.

In order to define the rôle of radiation therapy in the cancer effort, the CRTS first submitted a proposal to Dr. ENDICOTT, then Director of the National Cancer Institute, in August 1966. It was entitled 'A program for the optimal utilization of radiation therapy and the allied sciences in the treatment of cancer', and in it was suggested the creation of: (1) major radiation therapy centers, and (2) minor facilities at community hospitals. In March of 1967, our committee submitted a white paper to the NCI in which the requirements for major and satellite centers were spelled out. In October of 1968, the CRTS submitted a report to the NCI called 'A prospect for radiation therapy in the United States'. This 'blue book' made an attempt to define radiation therapy within the framework of the regional medical program concept. It described in some detail the present practice of radiation therapy and the need for three types of radiation therapy facilities, as well as the staff and facilities required in each of these types of facilities. Some 14,000 copies of this 'blue book' were distributed and it is now out of print.

At present the CRTS is completing a revision of the 1968 report, to express our present concept of the rôle of radiation oncology in integrated cancer management in the United States. This report expresses our opinion that the initial management decision is perhaps the most important single step in the treatment of cancer, and that this management decision should be both multidisciplinary and brought closer to the primary care level.

Finally, in an attempt to help identify the problems arising in the cancer center program and find solutions for them, our committee has joined with the Cancer Research Center Review Committee of the NCI to hold a number of workshops on this topic. These were relatively small working group meetings and were extremely useful in defining the multifaceted problems in the establishment of cancer centers. Unfortunately, it proved easier to define the problems than to find solutions for some of them; and further meetings will no doubt be needed for this purpose. A report prepared by Dr. WILLIAM POWERS and his group forms part of the minutes of our committee. It identifies the clear need for more data on the number of centers and types of centers needed, the impact such centers will have upon the community, upon biologic research, upon clinical cancer care and upon the national cancer plan. The value of planning activities needs further definition and the problem of inter-relationship of cancer centers with medical schools has to be clarified.

We see the rôle of the CRTS in the cancer center program as advisory to the NCI; we hope that we can present the point of view of the radiation therapy community. In order for our advice to be representative of the opinions and desires of our community, the CRTS is most anxious to get maximum possible input from all segments of the radiation therapy community; that is, both the academic and the private sectors. We believe there is a communality of interest and purpose in achieving one optimal level of care for the cancer patient, that all segments of the radiation therapy community will work together to establish a base upon which the interdisciplinary or comprehensive cancer center can stand.

Author's address: Dr. SIMON KRAMER, Thomas Jefferson University Hospital, 1025 Walnut Street, *Philadelphia, Pa.* (USA)

Front. Radiation Ther. Onc., vol. 8, pp. 29–35
(Karger, Basel and University Park Press, Baltimore 1973)

The Rôle of Radiation Therapy Related to Surgery and Medicine in the Past and Present

The British Experience[1]

S. DISCHE

Regional Radiotherapy Centre, Mount Vernon Hospital, Northwood, Middlesex

The concept of specialization in medicine has long been with us. Lord BACON, some 200 years ago, advised 'that medical men should make themselves proficient in physic by studying one disease at a time'. His advice was an encouragement to a Mr. JOHN HOWARD who established the 'Cancer Charity' at the Middlesex Hospital in London in 1792. It was the first of its kind in England and perhaps in the world. With the stated object of improving knowledge and methods of cure, a ward containing 12 beds was established for the care of cancerous paupers who were to stay until relieved either by art or by death. We can trace the history of specialized services for cancer patients in Britain from this small beginning.

During the 19th century the Royal Cancer Hospital was established in London and a number of other hospitals took some interest in malignant disease. Advances in management only follow the introduction of new methods of investigation and treatment. The microscopic study of tumours, anaesthesia and asepsis for surgery and the introduction of x-rays and radium at the end of the century heralded a new era in cancer treatment.

In the early years of the 20th century, a number of new research laboratories were established and also new institutions for the treatment of patients with malignant disease. The Radium Institute in London and the Holt in Manchester were founded for radium treatment. The Marie Curie Hospital was established for the treatment of gynaecological cancer in London in 1925.

As elsewhere in the world when radium was introduced it was used by the surgeons and by the gynaecologists and x-ray therapy was initially part

---

1   I wish to thank Sir BRIAN WINDEYER for his advice in the preparation of this paper.

of general radiology. Despite this, the distinct speciality of radiotherapy emerged in Britain in the 1930s in a way not seen elsewhere. This important development can be traced to a number of influences operating together.

One of importance was the National Radium Commission which was formed in the 1920s with a stock of radium raised by public subscription to celebrate the recovery of King George V from a severe respiratory infection. The loan of radium was subject to conditions to make sure of its proper use. The support of physicists was regarded as essential and all cases treated had to be registered and follow-up information supplied. Only large hospitals with adequately trained staff and facilities were in a position to use such radium. The commission established regional centres outside the London area usually in hospitals associated with universities. Full-time radium of-ficers were appointed in each to carry out the requirements of the commis-sion. It is of interest that the registration system for radium cases grew later into the national cancer registration scheme in use to-day throughout the country.

Another factor was the general awareness in Britain of the hazards associated with the use of radium and x-rays, and we were the first to estab-lish a national commission concerned with protection. The advantage of placing the use of such potentially dangerous methods of treatment in spe-cialized hands was obvious.

The cost of the increasingly more sophisticated apparatus, even in those days, was a considerable burden on those hospitals wishing to be equipped for radiotherapy. As a result of this, many hospitals were prepared to make formal arrangement for reference of cases for radiotherapy to another hospital which had the required equipment. In the radiotherapy departments so established, the case load made it reasonable to employ radiotherapists full-time in the field. It was also more diplomatic for a radiotherapist to communicate with surgeons and gynaecologists in other hospitals than to have a surgeon or gynaecologist at the central institution in this position.

The advantages of centralizing services for radiotherapy in establishing and improving methods of treatment were best shown in areas outside London where there was often just one major institution to serve a large area. Manchester, under RALSTON PATERSTON, established an international reputation and showed how a system of radiotherapy could be applied in the treatment of large numbers of patients.

The emergence of radiotherapy as a small but strong and distinct specialty was highly dependent on the presence of a small group of men of great ability. They established the radiotherapist as a clinician caring for patients and not as a technician completing a prescription for treatment. They produced well organized departments for the treatment and follow-up care of patients. A strong section of radiotherapy formed part of the Faculty of Radiologists established in 1939. It is this body that has acted as the official voice of radiotherapists in negotiations at a national level.

When, in 1948, the National Health Service was established, the pattern for radiotherapy adopted followed logically upon all the developments in the 1930s. In the National Health Service all consultants, regardless of specialty, have the same rank and the same pay-scale. This equality of status has certainly helped in the establishment of smaller specialties.

For the administration of the Health Service the country was divided geographically into regions each with a population ranging from 2–4 million. Responsibility for specialized services – for plastic, neuro- and thoracic surgery as well as radiotherapy – rested with the Regional Hospital Board and was organized on a regional basis.

In each region, the distribution of population and the pre-existing facilities have influenced the service for radiotherapy which has emerged. In some there is a large regional centre without any facilities in the remaining hospitals, in others there are small peripheral units linked with the main centre, while in yet others there are a number of distinct centres all quite independent. This latter pattern is seen in the four Metropolitan regions which serve the 12 million people in and around London. Our centre at Mount Vernon serves only the peripheral part of the North West Metropolitan Region, while the central area is looked after by radiotherapy departments in 1 post-graduate and 4 under-graduate medical schools.

Whatever the pattern employed, an essential part of the system is the 'peripheral clinic'. The consultant staff at the regional radiotherapy centre make regular visits to the district hospitals in the area served. In a district hospital containing, say, 400–600 beds a consultant radiotherapist will attend, often with a resident to assist him, for a morning or an afternoon each week. He will hold an out-patient clinic seeing 'new' and 'old' patients, and will visit the wards. Usually the radiotherapist is an accepted and full member of the staff of the district hospital. Over a period of years close personal contacts are made and collaboration over the handling of the various forms of malignant disease established. A majority of the patients selected for radiotherapy will attend the regional centre as out-patients but if they are unwell or if hospital in-patient care is required, then they are admitted to the wards at the centre. Some of the out-patients travel there using their own transportation but most are taken each day by the ambulance service free of charge. At the conclusion of treatment the patient usually remains in the care of the radiotherapist but he will attend the peripheral radiotherapy clinic at the district hospital for subsequent follow-up examination.

Every peripheral clinic does develop its own character and this, while it is greatly influenced by the radiotherapist holding it, is as much altered by the local conditions and by the personalities of the consultant staff at the district hospital where it is sited. At its highest development the clinic is the centre of cancer management in the district hospital and the radiotherapist advises on all aspects of care. Important as it is to advise where radiotherapy can be employed it is just as important that he encourages the surgeon to undertake a very radical operation or advises a general practitioner that no further treatment of any sort is justified in an advanced case and that the patient's best interests will be served by good home-care and the liberal use of narcotics.

This satisfactory picture, however, is not seen in every district hospital. Where a hospital is small and remote it is not possible for visits to be made weekly. The individual radiotherapist may not be prepared to advise outside the limited field of radiotherapy and that forceful individuality which is often the make-up of a successful surgeon may not enable him to take advice from any other discipline.

It is important at this point to mention that however tightly organized the radiotherapy service, it is the right of any doctor whether surgeon, physician or general practitioner to refer his patient to the radiotherapist of his choice. This is obviously easier where there are many therapists within access and, in the London area, a very considerable minority of patients are referred outside the arranged system.

I would like to discuss further the relationship between surgery and radiotherapy in our country. The association with the surgeons and the gynaecologists at the district hospital level is a very personal one. Problem cases may be seen together and, in some instances, combined clinics may be held if time permits.

At the regional centre or radiotherapy department of a teaching hospital, combined clinics are regularly held. An ear, nose and throat clinic exists in all and to this may be added clinics held in association with all the surgical specialties. In each particular specialty it often follows that one surgeon develops a special interest in the handling of malignant disease within his field of interest. Such men are prepared to take on the difficult and problem cases for surgery and are encouraged in this by their colleagues as well as by the radiotherapists. Often these combined clinics are held in the radiotherapy centre.

The description 'oncologic surgeon' now so familiar in North America is rarely heard in Britain. To most surgeons the word 'oncologic' is strange or somewhat suspect. The surgical specialties are well recognized in Great Britain. Ophthalmic, orthopaedic, plastic, neuromir, thoracic and ear, nose and throat surgeons all keep within their disciplines rarely straying outside and their territory is rarely ever encroached upon. However, urologists have not yet reached this position over the whole country and surgeons with a special interest in disease of the colon and rectum stay for the time being among the general surgeons. Specialization is essentially by anatomical system and an oncological surgeon who would cut across these established specialties would be out of place. It is relevant that the 'head-and-necker', so familiar in some parts of the United States, has never become established in Britain.

When we come to consider the relationship of radiotherapy to general medicine it is important to stress that the radiotherapist remains essentially a clinician. Several years of training in general medicine often precedes that in radiotherapy, and he is responsible for the medical care of those patients admitted to his beds in the wards associated with the radiotherapy centre, as well as those who attend as out-patients. Most spend part of their working day managing their patients with chemotherapy. The radiotherapist therefore covers part of the field of the medical oncologist as seen now in the United States.

There are now, in London, several special units for medical oncology but these do not exist outside the major teaching centres. In the paediatric field, tumours in childhood tend now to be referred to the specialist children's hospitals where there are also facilities for treatment of acute leukemia. For the large majority of patients with malignant disease the medical management is in the hands of the general physician (internist) and the radiotherapist.

The national policy for cancer services rests with the government minister responsible for the National Health Service. A 'Standing Sub-Committee on Cancer' on which sit leading members of the medical profession, including surgeons, physicians, radiotherapists and radiobiologists, plays an important rôle in the formation of policy. This body has recently reviewed the facilities for cancer treatment and has re-considered the place for oncologic centres on the European pattern. The final conclusion of the sub-committee was that there was a need for certain centres for the treatment of malignant disease where radiotherapists and research men would be joined by surgeons and physicians. The primary purpose of such centres would be for teaching and research, and they proposed only a limited movement of work in cancer from the general physician and general surgeon of the district hospitals. When the report was passed around the various professional bodies there was universal opposition to the scheme suggested and great exception taken to any diversion of patients with malignant disease to cancer centres. It has now been decided to undertake certain experiments only and, in four regions, pilot projects are proposed.

What are the disadvantages of centralization of cancer services?

Firstly, it is felt that the separation of a patient with cancer from his home district and hospital for a period of treatment which may be prolonged should be avoided if possible. The direction of all out-patients with cancer to attend a cancer treatment centre would mean an even greater burden of travel for the patient and his relatives and an even greater strain upon the ambulance service. The name of a cancer treatment centre would, if every case of cancer was referred to it, attract an ominous reputation. With all our optimism we must recognize that most major forms of cancer are still lethal and that the majority of patients so diagnosed will succumb within a period of time. Further, the cancer specialists in their cancer centre may become remote from the staff of district hospitals and a 'them' and 'us' situation arise. Relationships will consequently deteriorate and with it the care of patients. The general experience with cancer will be limited and the physicians and surgeons will be less able to cope with those previously unsuspected and urgent problems in malignant disease with which they will still be faced.

We feel that all these disadvantages are considerable and justify, at this time, the maintenance of our present system. Research into radiosensitizers, the chemotherapy of solid tumours and the immune responses in malignant disease, may lead to advances in management which will require some reorganization of services for the patients. We hope for a gradual evolution rather than dramatic change. We will certainly look for solid proof of benefit before establishing new institutions and re-distributing the available resources in the Health Service.

It seems, therefore, that organization for the care of the majority of patients with cancer is not likely to change in the near future. The feeling in Britain is that the centralization of the treatment of all cancer may lead to some increase in knowledge and advance in treatment, but beyond the present centralization of radiotherapy and the provision of some special centres and units, the disadvantages of complete centralization are too great.

Author's address: Dr. STANLEY DISCHE, Regional Radiotherapy Centre, Mount Vernon Hospital, *Northwood, Middlesex* (England)

Front. Radiation Ther. Onc., vol. 8, pp. 36–41
(Karger, Basel and University Park Press, Baltimore 1973)

Cancer Centres

Canadian Experience

R. J. WALTON

Manitoba Cancer Treatment and Research Foundation, Winnipeg, Manitoba

The development of cancer control in Canada has been guided by two complementary influences:

1. National correlation and assistance through the National Cancer Institute and the Canadian Cancer Society – both voluntary agencies.

2. Provincial legislation – health care being a provincial responsibility.

The National Scene

In 1931, a Study Committee on Cancer was established by the Canadian Medical Association to explore the possibility of developing on a national basis an organized attack on cancer. Representatives from each province, having discussed *inter alia* the place of professional education in relation to early diagnosis, the analysis of results of treatment, the availability of radium, and the means of encouraging cancer research, suggested that the most fruitful lines of attack would be through a programme of public and professional education and the development of a major research effort.

In 1935, His Majesty King George V, in commemoration of the 25th anniversary of his succession to the throne, consented to the inauguration of a national fund to be devoted to the campaign against cancer in Canada. The King George V Silver Jubilee Cancer Fund for Canada gave Canadians their first opportunity of contributing financially to the fight against cancer, an amount of approximately half a million dollars being raised.

In 1937, the study committee presented a brief to the trustees of the fund, pointing out the need for a national organization to supervise and coordinate all activities in the field of cancer. With the financial support of the fund, the Canadian Medical Association thereupon established 'The Canadian Society for the Control of Cancer' and this organization over the next 10 years received an annual grant from the fund, representing the interest on the capital sum. A dominion charter was granted to the society in 1938 which defined and further extended its responsibilities and through the years this society, now known as the Canadian Cancer Society, has continued to develop and expand its activities as a voluntary health agency in the field of cancer.

In 1947, at a national conference called by the Minister of National Health and Welfare, the National Cancer Institute of Canada was established. Its responsibilities included the support of cancer research, the dissemination of scientific knowledge relating to cancer and the correlation of provincial programmes against cancer. Over the last 25 years this scientific and professional organization has worked closely with the Canadian Cancer Society, itself essentially a voluntary lay organization, to develop a joint programme designed not only to instruct and support those active in the attack on cancer whether through patient care, research or education, but to assist and relieve those afflicted with the disease.

It is of interest to observe that while the Federal Government actively supported the establishment of both organizations and, in their early days, provided a substantial fraction of their operating funds, this evidence of interest has dwindled until at the present time the Canadian Cancer Society receives no government funds at all. Moreover, the relatively insignificant annual contribution of $250,000 received from federal sources over the past several years by the National Cancer Institute is now to cease entirely in spite of very strong representations. The contrast with the position in the United States of America is of interest. The two organizations, however, acting in close consort, to the extent of sharing senior officers and occupying joint premises, have continued to receive enthusiastic public support sufficient to enable them to carry out their programme without severe curtailment.

The National Cancer Institute of Canada, aware of the advantages of concentrating radiotherapeutic facilities in large, well equipped centres, published in 1950 a booklet entitled 'Minimum standards of radiation therapy centres' and followed this up in 1957 with a revision under the title of 'Standards for radiation therapy centres recommended by the National Cancer Institute of Canada'. These booklets stressed the desirability, particularly in a country large in area and relatively sparse in population, of concentrating personnel and equipment for the treatment of cancer in centres able to provide each patient with the modality best suited to his needs under the direction of skilled specialist care.

In general, the recommended pattern is in effect across the country with the exception of one province, and in 1970 the Institute felt that the time was ripe to issue guidelines for the establishment of what were called 'cancer control centres' upon the basis of efficient radiotherapy centres so established. This booklet entitled 'Standards for cancer control centres in Canada' discusses the underlying philosophy of such centres, their essential components and, with special reference to the Canadian scene, suggests means to achieve the stated objectives.

In principle, such a centre should: (1) bring the best possible care to all afflicted with cancer in all its stages; (2) add to the store of knowledge of cancer through co-ordinated basic, clinical and epidemiological research activities, and (3) provide teaching on all aspects of the disease and its treatment.

It will involve almost by definition, a university, a hospital, a major radiotherapy facility and an active division of the Canadian Cancer Society, but the frame within which these components are assembled may vary within fairly wide limits. For example, all may exist within a large university-hospital complex and work together as a cancer centre. On the other hand, it is possible to recognize a self-contained centre equipped with its own beds and facilities and relating to a nearby university.

Provincial Programmes

The establishment of radiotherapy centres has been fostered by the action of most provincial governments in setting up or recognizing, each in its own province, an organization with authority and responsibility in the cancer field. Such bodies, depending on their administrative structure, are known variously as foundations, commissions or boards. Their presence and activity has in turn permitted the evolution of cancer control centres upon the basis of radiotherapy centres already established.

For example, in Ontario in addition to the Princess Margaret Hospital (Ontario Cancer Institute) several other Ontario clinics have well integrated programmes. In Manitoba the Cancer Treatment and Research Foundation fulfils, with its university and hospital links, the criteria of a centre and will be described in more detail. In British Columbia a study just completed foresees a complete integration of cancer facilities on a province-wide basis;

while in Saskatchewan and Alberta, well integrated clinical facilities are now receiving the benefit of university affiliation. In the Maritimes, government-sponsored clinics now exist but it may be some time before they can develop to include the other components. In Quebec alone there is no organized control programme, each hospital providing what it considers appropriate facilities for radiotherapy.

The provision of health care is a provincial responsibility in Canada but its cost is shared between the provincial and federal governments, within the provision of the federal act. The financial support for a cancer control centre will clearly, therefore, derive from several sources: (1) federal government via health care and education funds; (2) provincial government via health care and education funds, and (3) granting agencies such as the National Cancer Institute of Canada, the Canadian Cancer Society and the Medical Research Council (this latter being federally financed to support research).

In essence, therefore, the cost of the education programme of a cancer control centre will be met through the budget of the affiliated university, the cost of health care will be met through normal health channels, while the cost of research will be covered by granting agencies with some assistance from the government.

A brief description of the Manitoba Cancer Treatment and Research Foundation may serve to put some flesh on the bones of the Canadian scene. Formed in the 1930s, the predecessor of the foundation, the Cancer Relief and Research Institute, was charged with responsibility for the provision and handling of radium. The need for welfare and public education services was soon apparent and the institute accepted the additional load. X-Ray departments were established in the Winnipeg and St. Boniface General Hospitals in the 1930s and these were taken over by the Institute in 1941 and 1954, respectively.

In 1937, the Provincial Cancer Registry was set up and now contains information on over 80,000 patients. During the same period a province-wide biopsy service was established. Like the therapy service, such diagnostic benefits were available to all Manitobans at no cost. In 1956, a nuclear medicine service was established in the two main hospitals.

In 1957, the Manitoba Cancer Treatment and Research Foundation was established to succeed the institute, while responsibility for lay education, patient welfare and the collecting of monies by public appeal were transferred to the newly activated Manitoba division of the Canadian Cancer Society. The foundation thereupon became a professional and scientific organization whose members are appointed by the government of the province. It maintains contact with the medical profession through a Medical Advisory Board also appointed by the government from nominations by organized medicine. It maintains a full-time salaried staff, the professional members of which hold appropriate appointments in the University of Manitoba and such hospital appointments as are necessary. The organization provides all the radiotherapy for Manitoba, 90% of the chemotherapy and a cancer consulting service in these two disciplines which is province-wide. Situated in the Health Sciences Centre, it has close links with the Medical College of the University of Manitoba and draws from the associated hospitals those services which it does not itself provide, notably surgery, pathology, diagnostic radiology and bed-accommodation.

The Manitoba Institute of Cell Biology represents the main research arm of the Foundation and is established by agreement with the University of Manitoba, each bearing one-half of the financial responsibility. With a present staff of 11 senior investigators, shortly to be increased to 25, the work of the institute proceeds on a firm clinical base. Nine of the present staff are clinicians, holding appointments in the Department of Medicine in the Faculty and being responsible for the treatment of patients by chemotherapy and immunotherapy. The addition of further investigators will provide greater breadth in the basic sciences.

The Physics Department, in addition to providing supportive services to radiotherapy has its own research programmes and operates electronic and mechanical workshops which are available to all hospitals in the area. It also provides for the provincial government a radiation protection service which exercises surveillance over all radiation producing equipment in the province. Through its physics department the foundation owns and maintains all nuclear medicine equipment in the main medical centres. The actual clinical operation in nuclear medicine was handed over to a joint university-hospital department 1 year ago, the foundation having assisted in the training of adequate professional and technical staff to carry on this work.

The Department of Epidemiology and Medical Statistics carries out research into the incidence of cancer in the polyglot population of Manitoba. It maintains the cancer registry and an abstract on all cancer patients in the main hospitals. It is also responsible for collecting and analyzing information derived from the province-wide cytological service.

The Department of Social Service, with the financial backing of the Canadian Cancer Society provide funds for cancer patients of limited means who may require assistance in such matters as travel, board and lodging.

The effort of the foundation in the field of education is exerted through university departments at the clinical and scientific level and directly at the appropriate technical and nursing levels.

While there is still much to be done, particularly in achieving the total integration of surgery, it is felt that at least a start has been made in honouring the principles enunciated by the National Cancer Institute as follows:

1. An interdisciplinary approach to the clinical, research and professional eduction components.

2. Total patient care, beginning with public education and extending through all stages of the disease.

Author's address: Dr. R. J. WALTON, Executive Director, Manitoba Cancer Treatment and Research Foundation, 700 Bannatyne Avenue, *Winnipeg R3EOV9, Manitoba* (Canada)

Front. Radiation Ther. Onc., vol. 8, pp. 42–48
(Karger, Basel and University Park Press, Baltimore 1973)

The Care of Cancer in the USSR

M. Lenz

Columbia Presbyterian Hospital, and Montifiore Hospital, New York, N.Y.

All care of cancer, as all medical work in the USSR, is controlled by the Ministry of Health. There are 16 ministries, one for each of the 15 republics and the chief ministry of Moscow which supervises the work of the entire USSR.

Each ministry has associated with it a scientific council, most of the members of which are doctors. The council suggests the medical policies, and these are then formulated into health laws and implemented by the administrative branches of the ministries.

Each Ministry of Health has a special cancer service which, in turn, has a few large central hospitals and institutes and a network of smaller peripheral institutions distributed throughout each republic. The administration of the oncologic service is centrally controlled and is divided geographically like other government services, i.e. into services of the republic, oblast (state), gorod (city) and smaller units including parts of a city (rayon). Each institution in these subdivisions is managed medically by its own director, but the director is responsible to and cooperates with the local chief oncologist, who represents the Ministry of Health.

The Rayon Oncologist

The chain of command of the oncologic service starts with this lowest link, the rayon oncologist. He is responsible (1) for cancer propaganda, arranging for lectures, exhibits, and other methods of cancer education of the laity, and (2) for cancer prevention – providing compulsory repeated health examinations of people with precancerous lesions or no evidence of cancer. At times large sections or whole towns may undergo such repeated health examinations so as to preclude the occurrence of neglected cases, not recognized until their cancer has become extensive. For these mass examinations the rayon oncologist gets temporary additional professional help, i.e. for cancer care or for referring the cancer patient elsewhere for further study and treatment. This referral may be to an oncodispensary or one of the larger central cancer institutes, since most of the rayon oncologists have only a small diagnostic office ('oncocabinet') for follow-up of cancer patients in their own district. A new cancer patient applying for the first time to a rayon oncologist is registered with him for life. Regardless of where the patient is treated thereafter, a record of follow-up is kept in the office of the first rayon oncologist, until the patient has died. This, then, is a permanent check on all later follow-up records from institutions in which the patient has been subsequently treated.

Oncodispensaries

One of the most important groups in the network of smaller cancer institutions is that of the 'oncodispensaries'. These are hospitals with from 30 to several hundred beds for surgical, medical, gynecological and other services, the number of beds depending on local requirements. A service for superficial radiotherapy and the usual laboratories for pathological and x-ray diagnostic services are provided. According to ZUBOWSKI, who supervised the construction and equipment of all oncodispensaries in the Russian SSR 5 years ago, there were 72 sanitary districts in the RSSR, each with an oncodispensary. In 60 of these oncodispensaries the radiotherapeutic equipment was modern, with fixed or moveable 4,000 Ci cobalt bombs. In the rest there were available mainly orthovolt x-ray and weaker cobalt bombs.

Admission of patients. Cancer patients may be sent to the oncodispensary by a rayon oncologist, or may enter it either directly through the polyclinic of the oncodispensary or, which is commoner, through one of the general polyclinics, that may be attended by any Soviet citizen. They are staffed by general physicians, specialists, and usually one or two doctors especially interested in cancer. To these special doctors are referred all patients in the clinic suspected of having cancer. If they agree and deem it advisable, the patient may be referred to the oncodispensary for further study and treatment, or be sent to one of the larger central institutes.

Treatment policies. The principles of treatment of patients who are taken care of in the oncodispensaries tend to follow a general outline arranged by the staffs of the larger central institutes depending on the type and stage of cancer. These outlines and plans of treatment, which are the result of a great deal of study and repeated trials, are not transmitted to the oncodispensaries until the testing staff has found them satisfactory. The conclusions as to treatment policies resulting from these tests are incorporated in form-letters. These are sent to all oncodispensaries from time to time and are, in general, followed meticulously. A certain freedom of action in their application, however, is at times permitted to qualified members of the oncodispensary.

Radiation protection. On only one point can there be no deviation from the postulated rules and principles – that is, the amount of protection from radiation used for the patient and personnel; these rules are strict and cannot be changed by the local authorities. Thorough protection from radiation is emphasized througout the USSR. Such protection requirements often necessitate special equipment and facilities. For instance, for insertion of intracavity gynecological radium, a special lead-lined chair is provided for the gynecologist and lead glass screens for the assistants. If the radiation quantity used in the patient is high, the bed patients are housed behind thick cement walls. Excretions are not allowed to escape into the general sewage system until their radiation activities have been markedly reduced by being kept in settlement tanks. The patient's linen is taken care of separately from the laundry of nonirradiated patients. However, these strict precautions are not observed if the radiation quantities are small.

The staff. Members of the medical staff of the oncodispensary have usually received their training in oncology in the larger central institutes. A general practitioner, surgeon, radiotherapist or other doctor will usually spend at least 3 years in such an institute before attempting to qualify as an oncologist.

Postgraduate and refresher courses and specialization are all directly controlled by the ministries of health. Most of the teaching centers are located in Moscow, Leningrad and other large cities, or within easy commuting distance. The postgraduate student is aided financially by continuance of his salary or grant of a stipend, and all expenses such as travel, lodgings and food are paid by the Ministry of Health. The refresher courses may last from a few weeks to several months, and often result in advancement in professional standing and economic status.

In addition to the ministries of health, there exist semi-independent academies of medical sciences which, like the ministries, may either belong to the health system of the entire USSR or be part of the local system of the individual republic in which they function. These purely scientific bodies do not have any legislative power, but are responsible only for research, which is done in about 28 institutes directly under the control of the academies. Many of these institutes are a combination of hospital services and laboratories. The hospital, however, will not treat average cancer patients but only those selected by the particular institute for its cancer research problem. Patients enter the research hospitals willingly, as they are conducted on a high medical level and their reputation is good. In these hospitals, new methods of diagnosis and treatment of cancer are investigated or developed; attempts are made to test, improve and standardize old methods, as well as to do pure research. At times, they may also do specialized teaching.

To be nominated, applicants for membership in the Academy of Medical Sciences must be less than 55 years old when nominated, must have made important contributions, and must have shown qualities of leadership. They are the élite and most respected members of the medical profession, and enjoy special economic and other privileges.

Though cancer research is carried out in all the academy institutes and in many of those more directly controlled by the ministry, each of these institutes, in addition, emphasizes one or another aspect of the cancer problem.

The *Gertzen Oncologic Institute*, RSSR in Moscow, is regarded as a model cancer hospital of the Russian Socialist Soviet Republic. It should be noted, considering the amount of radiotherapy conducted there, that although there were no physicists at the institute in 1959, by 1967 there were 10. They have a large animal house and another house for raising food for these animals, including special facilities where, for instance, they raise fresh winter grass.

There is also an outstanding viral and immunological laboratory. The large clinical material and experimental facilities provide good opportunities for teaching oncology, and the Gertzen Institute has become one of the best-known centers for postgraduate instruction of this specialty.

The impression of progress that I gained at the Gertzen Institute was corroborated by my visits to other institutions in Moscow, Obninsk, Leningrad, etc. Everywhere efforts were being made to modernize and improve cancer research, diagnosis and treatment. Old buildings were being replaced by new and larger ones, provided with better equipment and working facilities.

The Institute of Medical Radiology. Postgraduate teaching is done in other institutions, for instance the Institute of Medical Radiology of the Central Postgraduate School. This occupies a floor of the Botkin Hospital and is located next to the Gertzen Oncologic Institute. X-ray diagnosis, diagnostic use of radiation isotopes, and other subjects in diagnostic and therapeutic radiology are taught there.

The Institute of Experimental and Clinical Oncology of the Academy of Medical Sciences, RSSR, in Moscow, had the usual surgical, medical and radiotherapeutic services, but its particular interest was chemotherapy.

The radiotherapeutic service has physicists, radiobiologists and doctors who are particularly interested in radioactive isotopes.

In the Institute for Radiologic Research of the Academy of Medical Sciences RSSR, in Obninsk, the primary interest is radiation biology, as well as atomic and nuclear research. The institute is a $1\frac{1}{2}$-hour drive by car from Moscow. It consists of a clinical and an experimental section about 5 mi apart. According to Prof. ZEDGENIDZE, the Director in 1967, there was nothing here but virgin forest before building of the Institute was started in 1961. At the time of my visit 5 years ago this was an active town with streets, water supply, sewage disposal, electric power, homes, kindergartens, schools, a cinema and a restaurant. The entire population of the town worked directly or indirectly in projects related to atomic and nuclear research. The town is on a small river which supplies the atomic pile with water. The pile is located on one side of the city and, it is claimed, was the first pile to be used solely to produce electricity. Near it have been built institutes of physics, physical chemistry and applied geophysics.

On the other side of Obninsk there were, at the time of my visit 5 years ago, hospitals for clinical research and treatment of about 200 or more cancer bed-patients. This clinical section was directed by a hematologist especially interested in Hodgkin's disease. Only solid isotopes in closed containers were employed in this part of the institution. There were surgical, medical, gynecological, urological and radiotherapeutic services with beds for hospitalization of patients, as well as a small 'pensionat' or boarding house, solely for nursing care. Pathology and x-ray diagnosis were provided in the building.

The experimental section is devoted to animal and clinical research. Cancer patients requiring treatment with open isotopes are treated in this section. The animal house, I was told, contained 36,000 mice, rats and other small animals. All types of cellular, nuclear and other research on radiation changes in animals are done here. Radiation effects in genetics are being investigated in the Timofeyev-Ressovsky laboratories. In order to have a standard test object, Dr. Podsosov developed a special breed of rats ('August rats'), the physiology, chemistry and other characteristics of which have been studied and standardized.

The Scientific Research Institute of Roentgenology and Radiology, Academy of Medical Sciences, RSSR in Moscow, has about 450 doctors, biologists, physicists, chemists and construction engineers whose activities are directly or indirectly related to the care of cancer in the RSSR. All plans for buildings, equipment and standardization of diagnostic and therapeutic methods to be used in the RSSR are developed and tested in this institute. Only after these methods have satisfied the testing staff of the institute do they transmit their conclusions to the rest of the medical profession concerned with these particular diagnostic or therapeutic procedures.

The Scientific Research Laboratory of Proctology of the Ministry of RSSR in Moscow, has a rapidly growing 'in-bed' hospital service and ambulatory outpatient department. The service is devoted to care of tumors, cancer and precancerous lesions of the rectum and colon; colitis, including nonspecific ulcerative colitis; and to other inflammatory and ulcerating diseases of these organs.

The Leningrad Institute of Oncology of the Academy of Medical Sciences USSR, is located in Pesochnaja, in a newly-built complex of several 5- or 6-story structures, a $\frac{1}{2}$-hour electric train ride from the city of Leningrad. The institute has large clinical services in medicine, surgery, gynecology and radiotherapy, as well as a special building for experimental research.

In the research building are laboratories for experimental chemotherapy, immunology, study of animal strains, endocrinology, clinical cytology and physics. Considerable work in mammary, pulmonary, gastrointestinal, uterine and ovarian cancer is done here.

There is good, modern radiotherapy in a separate building with supervolt x-ray and cobalt-beam equipment.

A small department for orthovolt x-ray therapy and still lower voltages for skin and other superficial cancer has remained in the main building under the guidance of an experienced radiotherapist.

There is an oncodispensary in the Russian SSR at Sochi, a seaside vacation resort for Soviet citizens. Here are hundreds of sanatoria and rest houses that belong to individual workers' unions, who can send their members to Sochi for a free 3-week rest. This oncodispensary controls the cancer work in the city of Sochi and surrounding counties, and is connected with numerous local polyclinics, oncocabinets and other small diagnostic units from which their cancer patients are drawn.

The Ukrainian Research Institute for Experimental and Clinical Oncology in Kiev is directly under the jurisdiction of the Ukrainian Ministry of Health; it contains both experimental and clinical parts. In the research section they are studying cancer etiology, detection of cancerogenic substances in industrial enterprises, and the relationship of endocrine hormones to breast cancer. The transfer of leukemia from leukemic to nonleukemic mice by the use of RNA from leukemic tissues was demonstrated elsewhere. At this institute a similar transfer in rats has been performed.

The equipment includes such modern facilities as an electronic automatic counter for counting erythrocytes, leukocytes and cancer cells.

The clinical division has beds for cancer patients and an outpatient clinic. A large radiotherapy department includes supervoltage isotopes and cobalt treatment.

The Scientific Research Institute of Roentgenology and Radiology of the Ukrainian SSR is also in Kiev, and cancer treatment and research has been carried on there for years. Here, also, is the center controlling the various smaller cancer institutions in the Ukraine.

The Kiev Scientific Research Institute for Otolaryngology of the Ukrainian SSR has a large clinical division and a special 4-story building for otolaryngologic research. Many laryngectomies are performed here and research in various interesting (ENT) projects have been conducted here; such as the experimental production of pharyngeal cancer in rats.

Author's address: Dr. MAURICE LENZ, 1375 River Road, Apt. 2F, *Edgewater, NJ 07020* (USA)

Front. Radiation Ther. Onc., vol. 8, pp. 49–54
(Karger, Basel and University Park Press, Baltimore 1973)

On the Organization of Non-Surgical Oncology

Scandinavian Experience

J. EINHORN

Radiumhemmet, Karolinska Institute and Hospital, Stockholm

During the last few years, a relatively large number of investigations on the organization of cancer care has been presented in different countries and by WHO (table I). All of them emphasize the need for a special organization for cancer care. The technical report of the WHO [1966a] states: 'To deal with the cancer problem, the aim should be to establish a network of specialized cancer treatment centers.' This is agreed on in all the other studies officially published over the last 7 years by WHO and by the authorities responsible for cancer care in various countries.

There is also very close agreement on the functions of a cancer centre. These aims should be: (1) treatment of patients; (2) education and training

Table I. Governmental and WHO investigations on the organization of cancer management 1965-1972

The President's Commission; a national program	USA	1965
Technical Report No. 322, Cancer treatment	WHO	1966
Planning a radiotherapy department	WHO	1966
Hospital planning and administration	WHO	1966
Code de la Santé Publique; Centres de lutte contre le cancer	France	1969
Commission; Directorate of Health	Norway	1969
Department of Health; Cancer Advisory Subcommittee	Great Britain	1970
US Senate; special commission	USA	1970
The National Cancer Institute	Canada	1970
Socialstyrelsen	Sweden	1972
Reorganized	USSR	executed

in oncology, and (3) oncological research; development of methods for the treatment of cancer.

There is also close agreement on the allocation of cancer centres. In reports which deal with the problems of allocation, it is estimated that one cancer centre should be allocated for a population of 1–2 million people. In a population of 1,000,000 people, 3,000–3,500 new cancer cases a year may be expected. It is estimated that about 2,000 of these would be referred to the cancer centre. Only under special geographic conditions should cancer centres be established for less than 1,500 new cancer patients a year.

In all the national and international reports officially published over the last 7 years, there is very close agreement on: (1) the *need* for cancer centres; (2) the *aims* of cancer centres, and (3) the *allocation* of cancer centres; but the agreement is not complete on the most suitable *organization* of these centres.

There are two main alternatives for the organization of a cancer centre:

1. A separate and complete oncological hospital, with all the facilities for the treatment of cancer patients.

2. An oncological centre within a large general hospital – a nucleus specialized in oncological services, which has to rely on the various facilities of the general hospital for the total care of the cancer patients.

Another point of disagreement might be the internal organization within the oncological hospital or oncological centre.

In this paper, the organization of the non-surgical cancer care in Sweden and in the other Scandinavian countries is discussed.

In the Scandinavian countries, usually the same physician is responsible for radiotherapy and for all the other methods used in the treatment of malignant solid tumours except surgery. This organization might seem, here in the United States, strange to you and perhaps somewhat impractical; but it should be viewed against the development of cancer care in the Scandinavian countries over the last 50 years.

In Sweden, radiology was divided in 1917 into diagnostic and therapeutic branches, these two forming entirely independent and unconnected departments. Since then the Swedish radiotherapists have been trained in radiotherapy and oncology only. Beds have been assigned exclusively for radiotherapy since 1910.

Treatment at radiotherapy departments in Sweden has been cost-free since 1910 and so has the conveyance of patients to and from these departments since 1918. Facilities for following up patients were established at these departments in 1921 and, until today, 50 years later, mainly radio-therapists are responsible for the follow-up of cancer patients.

Every tenth year, when the king celebrates a round-figure birthday, a subscription fund is opened in Sweden, the money collected being used for any purpose the king considers most useful for the people. When Gustav V celebrated his 70th birthday in 1928, the fund was used to establish 3 radiotherapy centers in Sweden. These centres were and are independent departments within large hospitals, with their own beds and with an established, and in the country generally accepted, organization for the follow-up of cancer patients. The number of such departments is growing and the same type of organization has been established in Denmark, Norway and Finland.

By the time hormone therapy and chemotherapy were introduced, the radiotherapists in the Scandinavian countries were well trained in clinical oncology, with quite a large number of own wards and beds, and responsible for the follow-up of patients. It was taken for granted that they should assume responsibility for the use of chemotherapy, hormone therapy and other non-surgical methods of treatment in those solid malignant tumours, which were also treated by radiotherapy.

As outlined recently by the Swedish Medical Board [Socialstyrelsen, 1972] the organization of cancer care will be based on oncological centres within large hospitals.

Sweden is divided into 7 regions, each region having one regional hospital. Each of these hospitals will have one oncological centre serving on average a population of about 1,000,000. The oncological centre will have a nucleus consisting of a department of non-surgical oncology. The present regional departments of radiotherapy, after reinforcement of the expertise in internal medicine, will be converted into these departments of non-surgical oncology. Within the oncological centre there will be cooperation between the non-surgical oncologists and the organ-specialized surgeons. Surgeons, hopefully specialized in oncology, will be acting both within the oncological centre and within their surgical departments as urology, ear, nose and throat (ENT) surgery, thoracic surgery, etc. (fig. 1). Included in the oncological centre will also be departments of radiation physics and tumour pathology, a division for following up of patients and, if possible, also research laboratories.

The department of non-surgical oncology at a regional hospital will be very large and sub-specialization will be necessary. This sub-specialization can be either according to the treatment *methods* used or according to the *organ* of origin of the tumours treated. The sub-specialization according to

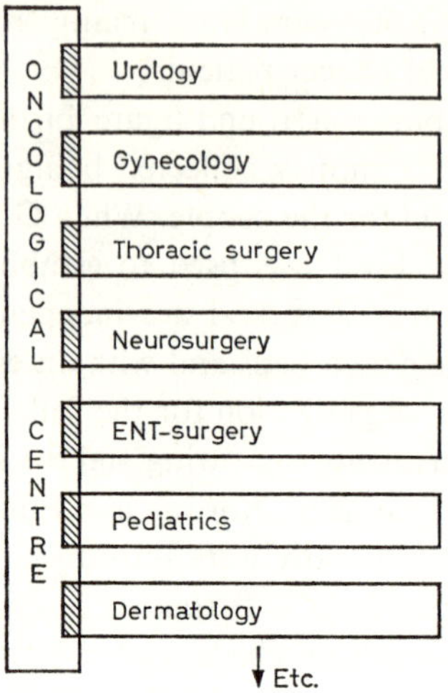

Fig. 1. Schematic organization of an oncological centre within a general hospital. ENT=ear, nose and throat.

methods would be in: (1) radiotherapist; (2) chemotherapist; (3) hormone therapist, and (4) immunotherapist; or various combinations such as: (1) radiotherapist; (2) medical oncologist, and (3) immunotherapist.

At the Radiumhemmet we have decided to sub-specialize according to organs. The main reason for this choice is that surgery is specialized in this way. We have brain surgeons, ENT surgeons, thoracic surgeons, urological surgeons, and so on. Sub-specialization of non-surgical oncology according to organs offers a very good basis for close collaboration between the non-surgical oncologist and the surgeon.

The organization at the largest of the regional radiotherapy departments in Sweden, the Radiumhemmet in Stockholm, is shown in figure 2. The department has 25 full-time physicians and a complete staff of more than 250. It has 132 ward beds, 450 visits a day for radiotherapy, chemotherapy, hormone therapy or follow-up examination and about 2,500 new cancer patients are seen annually.

At this department we have divisions of gynaecological oncology, urological oncology, etc. (fig. 2). The urological oncologists are responsible for radiotherapy, chemotherapy and, together with the urological surgeons, for hormone therapy in cases of urological tumour. Together with the urologists, the Urological Division of the Radiumhemmet has joint reception of patients, joint clinics, joint visits to the special urological wards and to the

RADIUMHEMMET, GENERAL DEPARTMENT, 1971

	BREAST GI TRACT NEURO.	THYROID PEDIATRIC	LYMPHOMA SKELETON	ENT LUNG SKIN	UROLOGY	GYNECOLOGY
OUT-PATIENTS no. visits/year	15,700	16,400	6,400	7,600	2,400	13,200
RADIOTHERAPY patients treated, %	40	6	10	30	14	
of beds, %	14	10	24	28	24	
COOPERATING DISCIPLINES	gen. surg. neuro-surg.	endocrin. pediatrics ped. surg. eye dept.	int. med. orthopedics	ENT dept. dermatology plastic surg. thoraxmed. thoraxsurg.	urology	gynecol. clinics
NO. PHYSICIANS	4.5	2.5	3	3	3	6
COMMON RESOURCES	clin. radiophysics, diagnostic and therapeutic isotope dept., megavoltage dept., chemotherapy ward, cytology, tumorpathology, radiation biology dept., follow-up product control, psychiatric care, research laboratories, oncologic library			The total number of out-patient visits at Radiumhemmet was 61,700. The total number of radiation treatments was 52,800		

Fig. 2. Internal organization of the radiotherapy department at the Karolinska Hospital and Institute (Radiumhemmet).

wards for urological oncology. The trainees at the Radiumhemmet are on a rotational schedule, serving at least 6 months at each division.

We do not know whether sub-specialization according to organs is superior to sub-specialization according to methods. Personally, I do not feel that in the future there will be much difference between the organization in different oncological centres. We must have close collaboration between radiotherapy and other types of non-surgical oncology. Basic research in chemotherapy and radiotherapy applies the same methods and is often conducted by the same people. Just how we sub-specialize in non-surgical oncology is probably not so very important, as long as we cooperate.

References

LLEWELYN-DAVIES, R. and MACAULAY, H. M. O.: Hospital planning and administration (WHO, Geneva 1966).

Central Health Services Council: On cancer organization. In report for the year 1970 (Her Majesty's Stationary Office, London 1971).

Code de la Santé Publique: Centres de lutte contre le cancer, section I-V, articles 312-325, annex I. (00000 Paris 1970).

Instilling fra utvalget for utarbeidelse av nye krav till utdannelse av strålterapi (00000 Oslo 1969).

National Cancer Institute of Canada: Standards for cancer control centres in Canada (National Cancer Institute, Toronto 1970).

National program for the conquest of cancer. 91st Congress, 2 nd session, US Senate (Senate resolution 376 and Senate report No. 91-1402) (US Government Printing Office, Washington 1970).

Socialstyrelsen:

The President's Commission on Heart Disease, Cancer and Stroke: A national program, vol. I and II (US Government Printing Office, Washington 1964-1965).

WHO: Cancer treatment. Technical report series No. 322 (WHO, Geneva 1966 a).

WHO: Planning of radiotherapy facilities. Technical report series No 328 (WHO, Geneva 1966 b).

Socialstyrelsen: Förslag till organisation av onkologin i Sverige (Socialstyrelsen, Stockholm 1972).

Author's address: Dr. JERZY EINHORN, M. D., Director, Radiumhemmet, Karolinska Institute, *Stockholm* (Sweden)

Front. Radiation Ther. Onc., vol. 8, pp. 55–62
(Karger, Basel and University Park Press, Baltimore 1973)

The Program of the Division of Cancer Grants of the National Cancer Institute

J. P. SAUNDERS

Extramural Activities, National Cancer Institute, Bethesda, Md.

Introduction

In the past decade, the National Cancer Institute has provided support for the development and operation of cancer research centers at educational and research institutions throughout the country. This activity has resulted in a great increase in cancer research, training and education in medical schools as well as in specialized cancer hospitals and research laboratories. Despite this, there still remains a need to create new centers and to strengthen and expand others, and it is for this reason that the President's initiative and the desires of the Congress have emphasized increased authorizations for centers. The general concept of a cancer research center is not something that can be created overnight by edict of the government or of any institution official. It is a concept that can only be realized in full partnership between the efforts of institutions and the medical community.

In 1955, the Congress appropriated sufficient funds for the first large scale attack on the cancer problem which launched the Cancer Chemotherapy National Service Center. That program taught us the procedures and techniques involved in organizing a large-scale government biomedical research effort based on the principle of cooperation and voluntary association of the National Cancer Institute with the scientific community.

On December 23, 1971, the President signed the National Cancer Act of 1971, which authorizes the Director of the National Cancer Institute, with the advice of the National Cancer Advisory Board, to plan, develop and execute an expanded, intensified and coordinated national cancer research program.

Under the act, authority is provided for support of appropriate man-power programs of training in fundamental sciences and clinical disciplines to provide an expanded and continuing manpower base from which to select investigators, physicians and allied health professions personnel, for participation in clinical and basic research and treatment programs relating to cancer including, where appropriate, the use of training stipends, fellow-ships and career awards.

Comprehensive Cancer Centers

The act provides for the establishment of 15 new centers for clinical research, training, and demonstration of advanced diagnostic and treatment methods relating to cancer.

Cancer center programs identified under section 408A of the National Cancer Act of 1971, hereinafter called comprehensive national cancer research and demonstration centers, ideally will have the following charac-teristics:

1. The center must have a stated purpose that includes carrying out of clinical research, training and demonstration of advanced diagnostic and treatment methods relating to cancer.

2. The center must have high quality interdisciplinary capability in the performance of diagnosis and treatment of malignant diseases.

3. The center should have or develop an organized cancer detection program.

4. The center must maintain a statistical base for evaluation of the results of its program activities. For this purpose records should be developed which will standardize disease classification to enable exchange of informa-tion between institutions.

5. The center should provide leadership in developing community programs involving active participation by members of the medical profes-sion practicing within the area served by the center.

6. The center must have a research base (fundamental and applied) and related training programs with an organizational structure which will provide for the coordination of these activities with other facets of the center program.

7. The center will participate in the national cancer program by inte-grating its efforts with the activities of other centers in an integrated nation-wide system for the prevention, diagnosis and treatment of cancer. For

this purpose the center must have sufficient autonomy to facilitate this function.

8. The center must have an administrative structure that will assure maximum efficiency of operation and sound financial practices. The administration should include responsibility for program planning, monitoring and execution as well as preparation of the budget and control of expenditures. Administration and management would include staff appointment and space allocation, the intent being that such a center will have the authority to establish the necessary administrative and management procedures for carrying out its total responsibility as defined in the criteria.

In addition to the comprehensive centers as defined above, the National Cancer Institute also supports specialized centers. Existing examples of such centers may be found in some of the radiation therapy programs which have been established over the past few years. Other examples may be found in center programs which are primarily concerned with chemotherapy of cancer. Existing center programs such as these may be considered part of the comprehensive centers program as defined above, if other qualifying criteria are met, the emphasis being the participation of such centers in programs of cancer detection, follow-up and evaluation, and the participation of physicians within the referral area in the programs of the center. The specialized centers may at some point form the nucleus about which a comprehensive cancer center may be built or it may continue to exist as a specialized center as a separate and distinct entity or as an integraetd part of a comprehensive center.

Funding

The National Cancer Institute will accept applications for support of all or part of the costs of planning, establishing or strengthening and providing basic operating support for existing or new centers: (1) for clinical research, training and demonstration of advanced diagnostic and treatment methods relating to cancer; (2) construction or renovation, and (3) patient care costs as are required for research.

Support by the National Cancer Institute will be accomplished by the award of grants following formal review as established by the National Cancer Institute and after favorable recommendation by the National Cancer Advisory Board. Support may be provided by one or more grants, the specific proposals in each instance should be submitted after consultation with the staff of the National Cancer Institute.

The initial support for new centers will be for a maximum of 3 years and may be extended for an additional period of 3 years following another formal review. This initial period of up to 6 years will be considered as probationary during which the applicant may demonstrate capabilities.

Since comprehensive clinical centers and program centers provide an established environment for productive work on cancer problems, the efforts of the Division of Cancer Grants activities in the National Cancer Institute will be to enhance the capabilities of existing centers and to establish new mission-oriented programs as a means of increasing benefits from these valuable resources.

The concept of a cancer center is a working together, an integrated effort on the part of all members of the medical community to gain certain objectives and to further the goals of cancer research for the community. It is a concept that requires that the operations of a cancer research center be 'open-ended' and, by its nature, multidisciplinary. The various components, each representing a particular program or programs, should be integrated to the extent that there is a coordinated approach toward solving cancer problems.

As can be seen, centers vary in their stage of development and, at the present time, three types of activities can be recognized. The first is the 'intradepartmental' program in which the attack on cancer is carried out in a single department or entity and is usually concerned either with a fundamental research approach or, if clinical, attuned to a single modality of treatment. Thus, we have radiation therapy programs and programs of chemotherapy in their own particular departments. Such programs of course, while valuable and contributing to cancer research, are limited in their scope and do not concern themselves with the broader aspects of the cancer problem.

The second type is the 'interdepartmental program' in which there is cooperation among several departments, permitting a multiprogrammed approach to cancer. Many of our leading clinical research activities are supported by this type of program and can lead to many sorts of collaborative studies both within and outside of a particular institution. Despite this enlarged scope, this type of program still does not address itself to the full breadth of the cancer problem in a medical community.

The third type of program is the comprehensive, institution-wide program which truly deserves the title of 'Cancer Research Center'. This perhaps is the ideal arrangement and often evolves gradually from the intra- and interdepartmental programs. Its main function is to provide a focus for cancer for the entire medical community. It should serve to provide a close coordination among fundamental scientists, clinical scientists, and practicing clinicians. It should provide such an integrated activity as to permit a rapid two-way communication between laboratory scientists and clinical scientists. In the medical community, it should provide leadership in the prevention, treatment and care of cancer, not by any bureaucratic system of control but by the intelligent practice of close community cooperation in the management of all aspects of cancer. In short, the National Cancer Institute seeks a system which will provide to the maximal extent possible a translation of research results into regular clinical practice, such that no citizen will be denied appropriate professional advice and care because of lack of facilities or knowledge.

Radiation Therapy Clinical Research Centers

This type of center continues to play a very important rôle in cancer management in many major clinical facilities throughout the country. Since it is well recognized that radiation therapy is essential in the management of cancer patients there is continuing interest in developing new radiation centers, particularly in medical schools. This facet of the radiation programs continues to grow, although somewhat slowly. At present 12 of these centers are being funded for a total of over $5,000,000. During this year, six new exploratory projects have been approved that could lead to expansion of existing radiation centers or the creation of new ones. Already a trend is detectable in that at some institutions ongoing radiation research centers are becoming the nucleus for the creation of comprehensive multidisciplinary cancer centers. It appears likely that in the future exploratory projects that originate in radiation therapy departments would be concerned with planning the development of this type of facility as a stepping stone to ultimate development of a comprehensive cancer center. This is a logical evolution since radiation therapists as a group are the physicians most closely identified with cancer in any major medical center.

Training in Radiation Therapy, Radiation Physics and Radiation Biology

Through past efforts of the National Cancer Institute the shortage of trained radiation therapists in the country has lessened. Following a policy of special emphasis of increased training in this field, 36 institutions are receiving support by means of training grants for a total amount just over $3,600,000. Through these grants approximately one-half of all physicians receiving training in radiotherapy at the present time are being supported by the National Cancer Institute. Despite these efforts there continues to be a critical shortage of radiation therapists as shown by a survey conducted by the Committee for Radiation Therapy Studies. It is unfortunate that most ongoing training programs have not sought support from sources other than the National Cancer Institute to continue operation. In view of the limited monies available for training such other sources of support must be sought to allow more new training programs.

A companion manpower problem is the need for training radiation physicists to provide the support required by radiation therapists in carrying out optimal forms of treatment. The American Association of Physicists in Medicine has shown great interest in this problem and grant proposals for training in medical or radiological physics can be anticipated in the future.

Cooperative Clinical Studies

The participation of radiation therapists in cooperative clinical studies continues to increase in a very gratifying fashion. The first such study initiated by the Committee for Radiation Therapy Studies, dealing with preoperative irradiation in lung cancer, has been completed. Other studies dealing with Hodgkin's disease and head and neck cancer are near to completing accession of patients into the studies.

More recently, 25 institutions agreed to form the Radiation Therapy Oncology Group (RTOG) to carry out cooperative clinical trials. This group has been reviewed favorably by the Cancer Clinical Investigation Review Committee and the National Cancer Advisory Board and is now receiving funds for its activities. At the present time this group is involved in projects studying irradiation of brain metastasis, split course of irradiation, and the effectiveness of hyperbaric oxygen and oxygen breathing in conjunction with radiation therapy for a variety of malignancies.

The creation of the RTOG is very encouraging since it will likely lead to a more meaningful dialog with other groups already participating in cooperative clinical trials under the aegis of the Clinical Investigations Branch. It is expected that the RTOG will come forth with additional protocols and, also, will help some other cooperative clinical groups in the preparation of protocols involving radiation therapy.

Research Grants

This category covers generally unsolicited research grants. At present about 60 grants of this type are being supported through this program. The total amount is just over $3,000,000. The scientific content of this category is broad spectrum, from the very basic to the quite applied. It cuts across the disciplines of physics, chemistry and biology. Basic studies include investigations into the molecular basis for radiation lethality and biochemical changes caused by radiation inactivation. Applied studies include computer analyses of tumor roentgenograms and optimizing automated radiation treatment planning. Physics studies include proton energy loss measurements. Chemistry studies include photochemistry of biologically important bases. Biology studies include RNA synthesis in mammalian cells after irradiation. The overall goal of this funding mechanism in the radiation program is to broaden the understanding of the interaction of radiation with biological material and to increase the impact of such information on the cure and prevention of cancer.

High Energy Studies

Another important goal in the radiation programs over the next few years is the assessment of the role of high linear energy transfer (LET) particle radiation in cancer therapy. There is already considerable experimental data suggesting that low oxygen tension renders mammalian cells less radiosensitive to the effects of γ-ray or û-radiation. Since most human tumors contain necrotic foci, it is very likely that at least part of the tumor population is hypoxic, which could account for many radiation failures. In fact it has been estimated that annually there are approximately 50,000 patients treated by radiation in whom the initial manifestation of recurring disease is at the site of the primary tumor. There is a growing consensus that many, if not most, of these local failures are due to the hypoxic tumor population which, if overcome, could yield dramatic improvements in cure rates. Excitement over high LET radiation is based on growing evidence that it may overcome the radioresistance of hypoxic tumor cells. A pilot study being carried out at Hammersmith Hospital in London appears to substantiate this for fast neutrons. In order to confirm these observations, if they are real, the National Cancer Institute is supporting several research projects in this country, using cyclotron-produced fast neutrons, that should lead to clinical trials in the near future. In addition, support has been provided for projects that studied the feasibility of designing a deuteron-tritium generator for the production of neutrons that could provide a clinically suitable source of neutrons for cancer therapy.

Another form of high LET particle radiation which seems to offer similar biologic advantage is negative Π-mesons. In collaboration with the Atomic Energy Commission the National Cancer Institute is funding the design and construction of a biomedical channel at the Los Alamos Meson Facility to study the possible clinical applications of this type of particle.

During fiscal year 1972 approximately $1,000,000 is being spent on high LET radiation efforts and it is anticipated that during fiscal year 1973 over $2,000,000 will be spent in this area.

Author's address: Dr. J. PALMER SAUNDERS, Ph. D., Associate Director, Extramural Activities, National Cancer Institute, *Bethesda, MD 20014* (USA)

Front. Radiation Ther. Onc., vol. 8, pp. 63–75
(Karger, Basel and University Park Press, Baltimore 1973)

The Planning of Cancer Centers

D. F. HERRING

Enviro-Med Inc. La Jolla, Calif.

Introduction

There is currently a great interest in planning for the development of cancer centers. Much of this interest has been stimulated by the passage of the National Cancer Act of 1971 which increased the amount of federal dollars going into the cancer field and raised professional and lay interest in the cancer problem to new heights. Although there is considerable interest in the concept of cancer centers, there is no well understood and commonly accepted definition of just what a cancer center is or what rôle centers are to play in helping to cope with and solve the cancer problem. Much of the uncertainty concerning this point has grown out of the way in which the term 'cancer center' has been used. For example, in fiscal year 1971, the year during which the National Cancer Act of 1971 was passed, the National Cancer Institute (NCI) funded 66 cancer center grants totalling $31,500,000 in a centers program which originated in 1961. Some institutions received two or three center grants, each of which supported different types of research activities. Some of these center grants are for broad, multidisciplinary clinical research programs, others are for highly specialized research programs in the preclinical or basic sciences. Now the term 'cancer center' has been incorporated into the National Cancer Act of 1971 to describe entities which are to conduct programs of clinical research, training and demonstration of advanced diagnostic and treatment methods relating to cancer. Thus, the term 'cancer center' has come to mean different things to different people. It is no wonder, therefore, at the uncertainty surrounding the use of the term 'cancer center' and the even greater uncertainty that exists concerning the planning of cancer centers.

Obviously, it is not possible at this time to remove all of the uncertainty concerning the definition and rôle of cancer centers and discussions concerning these matters will quite properly continue for some time. What is required, however, is to proceed, in spite of the uncertainty that does exist, with the business of improving and upgrading the quality of patient care, research and training in the field of cancer. This talk will, therefore, take a highly pragmatic approach to the problem of planning cancer centers.

The most important step in this pragmatic approach is to recognize that the *objectives of planning are to obtain funds for the support of cancer programs and to organize the programs so they make a demonstrable impact on the cancer problem in the region served by the center and wisely use the resources available to the center.* The objectives of planning, therefore, are not to prepare architectural plans, reports, etc., although these are important byproducts of the planning process.

In this paper, the sources of funds in the cancer field are briefly reviewed and then the steps and problems involved in obtaining some of these funds are discussed. The purpose of this discussion is to illustrate some of the important principles of planning. A review is given both of the planning process and of the conceptual framework for planning a cancer center. Finally, the reasons why it is important to plan a cancer center so that it is possible to demonstrate its impact on the cancer problem and its wise use of funds and other resources are discussed.

Sources of Funds for Centers

Potential sources of funds in cancer may conveniently be divided into 4 categories according to their purposes: research (both basic and clinical); training and education; patient care; and regional and demonstration programs. In each of these categories there are multiple potential sources of funds, as shown in table I. The division of funds in this manner has been to illustrate two very important principles in planning. Firstly, planning for a cancer center should take into account each possible source of funds so that a balanced base of support can be built up. Reliance on a single source of support can leave the center in a precarious position. Secondly, planning should assure that each source of funds is used in an appropriate manner because funding sources are becoming more specific as to what costs are allowable. For example, there is a trend for sources which pay for patient care to fund only those services directly related to the care of the cancer

Table I. Potential sources of operating funds to support cancer-related activities

Research basic and clinical	Training and education	Patient care	Network and regional programs
National Cancer Institute Grants: Research Program projects Cooperative programs Leukemia Support	National Cancer Institute: Graduate Training Clinical Training Research Fellowships Career Development	Private Patients Insurance Carriers Medicare Medicaid Patient Care Subsidies from State and Local Agencies	National Cancer Institute: Cancer Control Program Regional Medical Programs Office of Economic Opportunity
National Cancer Institute Contracts for Targeted Research	Area Health Education Centers (Bureau of Health Manpower Education)	Health Networks: Health Maintenance Organizations	Appalachia 202 Title 4A of Social Security Act
National Cancer Institute Grants-Contracts Organ Site Research	American Cancer Society		American Cancer Society Health Services and Mental Health Administration (Disease Control)
Institute of Dental Research, NIH			Charges to Recipient Institutions
American Cancer Society			314 (e) Neighborhood Health Centers
Other Foundations Gifts and Bequests			Office of Economic Opportunity Centers and Networks

patient and, conversely, sources of research funds are tending to pay only for research activities. In the past there has been considerable latitude in the use of funds allocated for patient care, research and training. This latitude will certainly cease, for all practical purposes, in the very near future as institutions receiving federal funds are being required to account more specifically for these funds. Failure to recognize this trend during planning could have a severe impact on the future financial stability of a center.

Cancer Center Grants

Having discussed the sources of funds available in cancer, it is important now to discuss the steps involved in obtaining funds. Only one source, namely grants for operational funds from NCI will be discussed here because they are the most important for a cancer center. Operational grants from NCI can be used for support in three main areas as discussed by SAUNDERS [6], ROBERSON [5] and EDWARDS [1]. Firstly, the centralized services such as experimental animal colonies, shared major equipment, and key scientific personnel; secondly, specific programs in training, basic research and clinical research, and thirdly, specific programs for regional demonstration and regional resources. Funds are also available for new construction and major alteration and renovation, as discussed by PRICE [4]. These are budgeted separately but are presently being awarded following the same review process as used for operating funds. Operational grant fund are important in the development of a cancer center as they can be used very effectively to marshal other resources available to the center. Therefore, the remainder of this paper is keyed to the planning process as it relates to NCI funding.

Review Process for Center Grants and the Importance of Planning

Figure 1 is a simplified diagram showing the relationship of NCI to other government organizations and the peer review groups. This figure is useful in explaining the review and funding processes. As you know, the

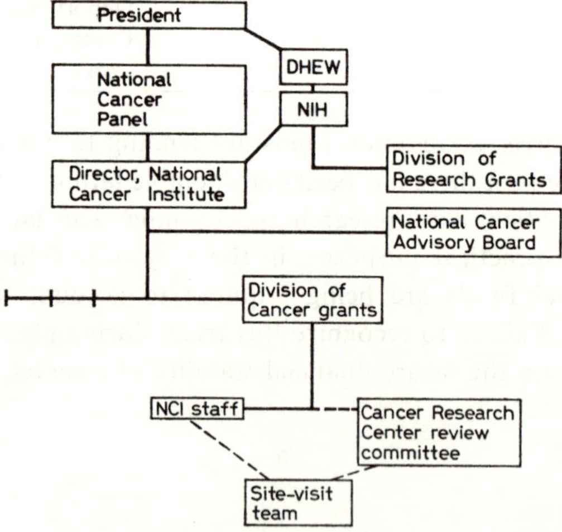

Fig. 1. Simplified diagram showing the relationship of the National Cancer Institute (NCI) to other organizational activities. See text for explanation.

National Cancer Act of 1971 created a 3-man committee, presently chaired by Mr. BENNO SCHMIDT, through which the NCI director, Dr. FRANK J. RAUSCHER, reports on management and budget matters to the president. The budget is reviewed by the National Institutes of Health (NIH) and the Department of Health, Education, and Welfare (DHEW), but they do little more than simply comment on it. NCI continues at the moment to follow the personnel policies, contracting mechanisms, and auditing and grants management procedures of NIH.

The National Cancer Act of 1971 also replaced the National Advisory Cancer Council with an enlarged National Cancer Advisory Board, which advises the director of NCI on policy matters. The board consists of 23 members, appointed by the president for 6-year terms, many of whom have distinguished records in cancer research.

Within NCI there are 4 divisions. One of these is the Division of Cancer Grants, headed by Dr. J. PALMER SAUNDERS. This division administers the operational grant funds. A Cancer Research Centers Review Committee (CRCRC), whose members are appointed by the director of NCI on the recommendation of Dr. SAUNDERS, has the responsibility for peer review of center grant applications.

Briefly, the funding mechanism works as follows. The applicant institution prepares a grant request and submits it to the Division of Research Grants of NIH which, in turn, sends it to the appropriate individuals at NCI. There is a technical review by the NCI staff and then the CRCRC arranges for an *ad hoc* committee to conduct a site visit as discussed by JAY [2]. Site visitors study the grant application and question members of the applicant institution in detail. On the basis of information thus obtained, the site-visit committee recommends approval or disapproval to the CRCRC along with a funding level and priority (if approved). The CRCRC may or may not modify the recommendation and then submits its recommendation to the National Cancer Advisory Board through the Division of Cancer Grants and the director of NCI. After approval by the board, the NCI staff determines the level and timing of funding after reviewing all approved grant applications and budget limits for programs.

The important point to be made concerning the review process is that while NCI staff has the ultimate responsibility for approving or disapproving grant requests and setting the levels of funding, it is required by law to use a peer review system in making these decisions. As is well-known, the NCI Division of Cancer Grants does not simply pay lip service to peer review – it relies heavily on the peer review system!

It is important, therefore, to determine as a practical matter how this combined staff-peer review decision-making apparatus functions. In principle, the site-review committee, the CRCRC, the National Cancer Advisory Board, and the NCI staff are all guided by criteria which have been developed over a period of some time and are contained in various NCI publications. These criteria are continually reviewed and changed, from time to time, as necessary.

From our experience, however, it appears that the overriding consideration is that the peer review system responds in a perfectly human way to the ever-present shortage of available funds by looking for ways to decrease the dollar level of the grant request or for bases for recommending disapproval. The site-review committee, therefore, searches for weaknesses in the grant request. Often a weakness in one area strongly influences a review committee and colors its view of the grant application as a whole.

Citing our own experience in working with institutions submitting this type of grant request, it appears that the site-review committee looks carefully at the following factors:

1. Scientific distinction and coherence of existing and proposed programs.

2. Scientific competence of program director and staff.

3. Administrative competence of program director and staff.

4. Degree of commitment from parent institution(s) with tangible evidence of support.

5. Clarity of statement or program objectives and adequacy of planning for meeting these objectives.

6. Suitability of organizational structure for attaining objectives.

7. Detailed justification for the amount and timing of funds requested and relationship to detailed programs.

8. Adequacy of planning for cooperation with other centers and best use of regional resources.

Accordingly, in order to meet the planning objectives, the planning process must be conducted in such a manner as to place the applicant institution in the strongest possible position to defend its grant application and to achieve credibility. This means that the planning should begin before submission of the operating grant application and the applicant institution should be thoroughly prepared for the site-review committee.

Clearly, planning itself cannot help the applicant institution where the scientific merit of programs and the competence of the program director and staff are concerned. The applicant institution either has qualified investigators or it does not. If it does, the planning process can proceed in an orderly fashion. If it does not, even an infinite amount of planning will not get the proposed program funded. Consequently, before beginning the planning effort, the applicant institution should satisfy itself concerning the competence of the program director and investigators responsible for the proposed center programs.

The planning process can greatly assist the applicant institution with all other factors given above. It can, for example, assist the program director and his staff with the development of an administrative program. Planning can provide the information upon which arguments for a greater degree of commitment from the parent institution can be based. Planning can assist the program director in clarifying the statement concerning the program objectives and can assist him in laying out the manner in which the objectives are to be obtained. Planning can analyze the suitability of various organizational structures for the cancer center and can evaluate their adequacy for reaching the objectives of the cancer center. Planning can provide an analysis of the overall funding requirements, can provide a detailed justification for the amount and scheduling of funds required for the development of the center, and can relate the funding request to the individual program requirements. Finally planning, when conducted with the proper degree of sensitivity, can be immensely valuable in obtaining the cooperation of other cancer programs in the region to provide the best utilization of the total resources of the region.

The Planning Process

Planning is a process which has two products. One product is the administrative and operational structure of the center. During the planning process, successful and cohesive working relationships should be formed between the potential participants in the cancer center in such a manner that these relationships can be carried over to the actual operation of the center after it is funded. The second product is the plan itself.

This plan must, of necessity, be tailored to fit the specific needs of the institution and thus no universally valid recipe for a planning process can be given. It is possible, however, to describe a general conceptual framework for planning, and this is done below by first describing the components of the plan, and then describing the steps for developing that plan.

Components of the Plan

The plan itself consists of several interrelated components, each of which should be stated for appropriate stages of development of the center. These are:

1. *A clear statement of the objectives* of the center indicating what the establishment of the center is expected to accomplish.

2. A *description* and *justification* of each program to be conducted under the aegis of the center. These programs can be grouped according to clinical care, clinical and basic research, training and education, and regional resources and demonstration.

3. A *definition* of the needs of these programs in terms of staff, space, special equipment, patients and other resources.

4. An *administrative and operational structure* that is adequate to ensure that the objectives are reached and that mutual support and interaction will occur.

Planning Steps

The plan components given above are time-dependent and are strongly correlated with one another. Thus, one component cannot be developed independently of the other. For example, the objectives of the center cannot be stated independently of the programs required and these must, in turn, be analyzed with respect to the availability of the resources required, the administrative structure and so forth. The planning process often tends to be an iterative one in which various alternatives for each component are considered until a matching set comprising a realistic plan is found. The steps outlined below are designed to minimize the iteration in planning and to produce the two products, namely the administration and operational *structure* and the *plan* itself, with a minimum of effort. The steps are as follows.

1. Organize a planning committee with a chairman who reports to either a dean or vice president. The committee should have sufficient representation to ensure that the group includes all necessary viewpoints and enough of the power structure to ensure that its recommendations are likely to be adopted by the institutions concerned. Ideally, the chairman should be a suitable candidate for the position of director of the cancer center, but this is not essential at this point in the planning process.

2. Obtain financial support for the planning committee to conduct a defined planning program. This support, which can be obtained from the institution or from an NCI exploratory grant, as described by WALTER [7], will enable key personnel to devote adequate time to the activity, and will enable consultants to be provided if desired.

3. Determine the present status of cancer-related activities in the institution and in the region and catalog these activities in a format suitable for use in the planning study.

4. Determine potential participants in the cancer center and involve them in the planning process in an appropriate manner.

5. Select a scientific review panel from members of the planning committee. This panel should be given the responsibility for evaluating the scientific merit of each program proposed for the center. Programs of marginal or questionnable merit should be excluded from the center by the planningcommittee chairman on the recommendation of this panel.

6. Formulate simplified alternative models for the cancer center at a suitable point (10 years) in the future. These are self-consistent and justifiable conceptual models which cover the spectrum of center types with respect to overall objectives, regional involvement, program size and content, resources required, administrative structure, etc. These models are idealized in the sense that their development from the current status is *not* considered in their formulation. On the other hand, they must be realistic in terms of the pecularities of the region to be served by the center, and the NCI funding policy trends. They are developed as an exercise to educate the planners concerning the way in which the components of centers relate to one another for each type of center and to form a basis for selecting a target center concept. Each alternative model should be described in writing with an organizational chart and quantitative estimates for patient load, staff, facilities, budgets, etc.

7. Select one of the above alternatives, or a modified version, as a target center. The selection should be based on the planning committee's judgment of the feasibility of attaining the target center in view of the economic and political realities peculiar to the institutions and individuals involved in the planning and in the region. The selection must be a matter of judgment since there is no other way in which these realities can be factored into the development of a center. The judgment is most likely to be realistic and practical if it is made by an informed group considering a well defined target center concept which is provided by step No. 6 above.

8. Formalize the status of the cancer center within the institution and select a director, scientific review panel and administrative system for the center. The director may or may not be the planning committee chairman and the scientific review may or may not be the same as that selected from the committee. The administrative system should be capable of evolving into that of the target center concept selected in step No. 7 and should enhance working relationships developed thus far in the planning process. The planning committee may be replaced by the operating structure at this point, since the decisions as to the context of the center will then have been made, and the remaining detailed decisions on the content of the center are best made by those who will be directly responsible for the eventual operation of the center.

9. Develop an overall schedule for the evolution of the center from the present to the target center concept. The schedule should be optimized with respect to funding cycles so as to minimize delay in the initiation of the centers program. New program areas to be included in the center and their schedules should be approved by the scientific review panel and the center director. Individual schedules should be prepared for each of the program areas of clinical care, clinical and basic research, training, education and regional resource and demonstration. The individual schedules should include submission dates for grant applications required to obtain funding for each program area. The overall schedule should be approved by the director, and the applicant institution and should have the endorsement of all others who are to be involved in the center development.

10. Develop the resource requirements as a function of time for each program area. These requirements include patients, staff, space, equipment and funds. Each of these requirements must be carefully analyzed with respect to resource availability.

11. Develop the cancer center plan and documents to justify and support that plan, and NCI grant requests for funding. The plan should be concise, easily readable and should encompass each component previously mentioned. Detailed justification for funding support, staffing, facility requirements, architectural plans, etc., should be presented in separate reports appended to the plan. The plan should, of course, be supportive of and consistent with grant applications submitted to NCI. It may be necessary to submit the grant request to NCI before the plan is complete in all of its details in order to meet deadlines established by NCI. In this case, the detailed plan should be completed before site-review so as to place the applicant institution in the strongest possible position to defend the grant application.

As can be seen, this process produces a workable administrative *structure* for the center in a logical and orderly fashion. The *plan* is also developed systematically with a minimum of iterative steps.

Impact Demonstration as a Planning Objective

The second objective of planning is concerned with the demonstration of the impact of the center on the cancer problem and the judicious use of funds and resources available to the center. The center should not only be able to demonstrate that it is achieving its objectives, but also that the NCI dollar is being used to marshal the resources of the community, to attract other support from both private and federal sources, and to upgrade the quality of care for the cancer patients in the region served by the center.

This planning objective is related to the need for continuity of funding for the cancer center over a period of years. Continuity of funding is important, not only because results of scientific programs cannot be evaluated in periods of less than 5–10 years, but also because medical schools are not going to want to make the substantial investment required to initiate a cancer center if the research and core activities of the center funded by NCI grants do not have a reasonable chance for continuing financial support.

The availability of grant funds for any given cancer center is related to the budget for the 'centers' program within NCI which is, in turn, directly related to the total NCI budget. As a general rule, it could be said that the larger the NCI budget, the more money that will go into cancer centers in the form of grants and contracts.

There is presently a need for more money in the centers program as evidenced by the fact that there are many center grant applications currently approved but unfunded. As more and more institutions become involved in the development of cancer centers, the demand for federal monies for cancer will continue to increase. Judging from the interest in centers evidenced at this meeting and at other meetings, this growth in demand is likely to increase much more rapidly than the supply.

Ultimately, the amount of money available to NCI is determined by Congress. Congress authorizes levels of funding for all national programs in accordance with national goals and priorities as determined through hearings and the political realities of the times. As Congress considers the appropriations legislation for the next fiscal year and the authorization and appropriations legislation for the fiscal years beyond 1974, it will certainly review the promises and statements that were made in the hearings held in connection with the formulation and passage of the National Cancer Act of 1971. These hearings and articles in the press lead one to believe that Congress expects one of two things to happen in the next few years: either a dramatic breakthrough in the basic sciences or a demonstration of the beneficial impact of cancer research on patient care throughout this country.

In this regard, the visibility of a center program could be an essential factor in establishing the credibility of an expanded NCI centers program. This credibility could in turn be crucial in obtaining funds at a level to assure that the center program can meet the needs of the country. Therefore, the planning process for each center should study the ways that the center can demonstrate that it is meeting its research objectives, that it is having a favorable impact on the cancer problem, and that it is wisely utilizing the funds and other regional resources available to it.

Two key points can be derived from the above discussion. The first is that the visibility of a center program must be achieved at the congressional level which is in turn achieved at the patient-voter level. As mentioned above, appropriations for these programs are set by Congress, and Congress consists of and is elected by cancer patients and potential cancer patients. Recent history has shown that Congress no longer has any difficulty in making major cuts in funds for domestic programs that fail to meet their objectives and do not directly benefit an identified need in society. Therefore, the effectiveness of the center must be visible at the congressional and patient-voter level. This would appear to be the best way to insure the continuity of funding for the cancer center.

This brings us to the second point – the visibility needed to assure the continuing funding of the center program must involve full integration of the private physician and the community hospital into the center program. One of the best ways to reach the patient-voter is through the private physician who serves as the point of entry for most cancer patients into the cancer care system. It is he who often makes the initial, crucial decisions concerning the management of the patient's clinical problem. Involvement of the private physicians in the center program is therefore in the best interest of the patient as pointed out by MARTIN [3] and also is of great importance in assuring the continuing financial support of the center. The relationship of the center to the private physician and community hospital should, therefore, not be neglected in the planning process. Particular attention should be paid to this point, especially since the peer review system is under the complete control of academic medicine and the private physician is very much aware and apprehensive of this fact.

Summary

In summary, the objectives of planning for cancer centers are to obtain funds for the operation of the center and to develop a plan for assuring the continuing support of the center. The planning process should, therefore, be conducted to place the applicant institution in the strongest possible position to defend the grant application at the time of peer review and to develop the center programs in such a manner as to make a demonstrable impact on the cancer problem in the region served by the center and to show that all resources available to the center are being wisely used. A conceptual framework for planning has been outlined which produces both an administrative structure for the center and the plan itself. These are important products of the plan process in that they provide the essential elements for defense of the grant application.

References

1 EDWARDS, M. H.: Role of the cancer center in training. Cancer, Philad. *29:* 889 (1972).
2 JAY, G. D.: Review and evaluation of cancer research center grant applications. Cancer Philad. *29:* 896 (1972).
3 MARTIN, L. R.: The primary physician and the cancer center. Cancer, Philad. *29:*902 (1972).
4 PRICE, S.: The National Cancer Institute Construction Grants Program. Cancer, Philad. *29:* 894 (1972).
5 ROBERSON, W. M.: Current National Cancer Institute Center Programs. Cancer, Philad. *29:* 887 (1972).
6 SAUNDERS, J. P.: The role of the National Cancer Institute in the development of cancer centers. Cancer, Philad. *29:* 882 (1972).
7 WALTER, W. A.: Planning for cancer centers. Cancer, Philad. *29:* 891 (1972).

Author's address: Dr. D. F. HERRING, P. O. Box 2324, *La Jolla, CA 92037* (USA)

Front. Radiation Ther. Onc., vol. 8, pp. 76–80
(Karger, Basel and University Park Press, Baltimore 1973)

The Joint Center for Radiation Therapy

A Multihospital Radiation Oncology Center

S. HELLMAN

Department of Radiation Therapy, Harvard Medical School, Boston, Mass.

As a prelude to a description of our efforts at the Joint Center for Radiation Therapy, it seems pertinent to inquire as to the objectives of a cancer center and the role of radiation oncology in achieving these goals. Obviously, the patient should be availed of that management most likely to achieve cure, long-term control, and/or palliation of the disease. Such care must be available to all regardless of economic, social or geographic considerations. There must be effective use of skilled, highly-trained personnel, sophisticated equipment and facilities. An active training program for expanding our limited personnel resources must be fostered. Finally, the activities of the center should be compatible with active clinical and/or basic research. This requires that maximum information must be derived from all patients. Cardinal to the function of the center must be the rapid translation of research advances to clinical application. The following will describe our attempt to meet these goals in a multihospital medical school setting.

The Joint Center for Radiation Therapy was organized in 1968 under the auspices of the Harvard Medical School to provide modern, comprehensive radiation therapy as an integral part of the management of patients with neoplastic disease at its then four member hospitals (the Beth Israel Hospital, the Boston Hospital for Women, the New England Deaconess Hospital and the Peter Bent Brigham Hospital). Since that time, the member hospitals have been expanded in two categories. The Children's Hospital Medical Center has joined, bringing the number of full members to 5. In addition, a new category of associate membership has been made for hospitals requiring only limited use of the joint center with the Faulkner Hospital being the first member to assume this rôle.

The *Joint center* provides sophisticated and comprehensive radiation oncology within the framework of a general hospital. A coordinated program in radiation oncology exists in which patients from any of the hospitals receive care, emphasizing those personnel and facilities within the center which are best suited for them, regardless of their hospital of origin. Thus, patients have access to the radiation oncology resources of all of the member hospitals and unnecessary duplication of personnel or facilities is avoided. The *Center* has grown in the 4 years of its existence so that it is now the largest radiation therapy center in New England.

There is a department of radiation oncology at each of the hospitals, these being divisions of the Joint Center for Radiation Therapy. All staff members have privileges within all of the hospitals. The senior staff members have a primary base of operation, allowing them to identify with that hospital staff. The junior staff, residents and technicians rotate through the different units. This fosters uniformity of treatment philosophy, and technique. The identification of a unit of the center with a permanent senior staff member within each hospital promulgates acceptance within that hospital of the radiation oncology team. Close working relationships with other physicians foster active participation by the radiation oncologist in *initial management decisions* – often the most important therapeutic maneuver. If we are to provide optimal care for patients, decisions with regard to therapeutic modalities must be multidisciplinary, combining the knowledge and skills of all cancer-related disciplines. Each division of radiation oncology actively participates in the multidisciplinary conferences, rounds, and all other functions of the hospital in which they reside. Thus, the divisions of the Joint Center for Radiation Therapy function in this setting very much like any of the other major clinical departments within the hospital. In addition, they also function as components of the Joint Center for Radiation Therapy. The center has uniform treatment policies. a common approach to management problems, common physics and technical staff, one system of records and a single tumor registry. The total facilities of the joint center, regardless of location, are available to patients from all hospitals and to staff radiation oncologists practicing in any part of the center.

In order to integrate and coordinate the operations of the center, all of the professional staff members of the Joint Center for Radiation Therapy meet at least once a day in formal conference. Patient management problems are presented at these conferences so that expert consultation can be given within the center. Further, general treatment protocols are evolved in the same fashion as would be true if the center had all of its facilities within one geographic location. The center attempts to provide all of the advantages of a large radiation center in a setting of close personal attention, cooperation, and high level of general medical care characteristic of the university hospital.

All of the cooperating hospitals have a formal area designated as the radiation oncology department administered by the Joint Center for Radiation Therapy. These contain, at the least, the physicians' offices and secretarial support, palliative therapy devices, examining rooms and follow-up facilities. In some, this includes major supervoltage radiation therapy devices, machine and electronics shops, a radiation therapy simulator, computers, etc. Unnecessary duplication is avoided and facilities are used to complement each other. Again, patients receive that portion of their therapy at whatever location is best suited for them, regardless of the hospital of origin. However, it is attempted to distribute physical facilities in a fashion most appropriate for the individual hospitals. One example of the common sharing of expensive physical facilities includes the Treatment Planning Center at the Boston Hospital for Women. Here, all patients receive their treatment planning. A majority of patients go to the planning center for at least one visit. Body contours are recorded, the treatment plan is computed, the treatment technique is rehearsed on the radiation therapy simulator, and beam modifying and immobilizing devices are custom-made for patients. When this is completed, the plans and devices are forwarded to the hospitals best suited for that patient's treatment. Other examples of specialized shared facilities include the electronics shop at the Beth Israel Hospital and the 12 MeV linear accelerator at the Peter Bent Brigham Hospital which is available to all patients whose treatment involves the use of high-energy electrons. There is a central tumor registry for all patients receiving radiation therapy. The charting and recording system is identical and the data bank is common.

In 4 years of operation, the number of new cancer patients being treated per year by the radiation therapy services within the hospitals has grown from about 600, before the joint center started, to the current level of approximately 1,700. The number of staff radiation therapists has increased from $2\frac{1}{2}$ in 1967 to 9 in 1972. The radiologic physics staff has increased from $1\frac{1}{2}$, before the development of the department, to 6 professional physicists as well as a large number of other support personnel involved in the technical considerations of radiation oncology. An active residency program has been formed so that there are now 9 residents in radiation oncology training at the Joint Center for Radiation Therapy. In cooperation with the Harvard School of Public Health, a graduate program in medical radiological physics has been developed. This leads to either a master's or Sc. D. degree and currently has 5 students. A radiation therapy technology training school has been formed with 7 students. Physical facilities include one 12 MeV linear accelerator, three 4 MeV linear accelerators, one cobalt-60 unit, a variety of orthovoltage and superficial units, a large supply of interstitial and intracavitary isotopes. In addition, we have the *Treatment planning center* which includes computer facilities, a radiation therapy simulator, a mould room and machine shop.

The *Center* has its research activities housed in the Shields Warren Radiation Laboratory. Currently, there is active research at both the basic and clinical levels. Some clinically-related investigations include radiation-drug interaction, antigens associated with Hodgkin's disease and late stromal effects of radiation. Important is the ease with which clinical observations can stimulate laboratory investigation as well as the rapidity with which research findings can be incorporated into the clinic. This is fostered by active participation of the clinical staff in the research activities of the department.

One might ask if this model is applicable to other centers in other locations, or does it represent a development possible only because of unique local arrangements. This is difficult to answer. Clearly, such an organization requires close cooperation by member hospitals with a minimum of interinstitutional friction, competition or jealousy. The director must have the complete confidence of all of the hospitals; his position should be of the same level as that of the chiefs of other services at each of the hospitals. The department within the hospital should be considered the same as other departments. Harvard Medical School has been very helpful in developing the Joint Center for Radiation Therapy. It acts as a supra-hospital unifying influence and gives further structure to the combined department.

If such a joint center is to work, then each hospital must make an appropriate commitment of resources and finances but should expect an appropriate return in services rendered. The hospital staff must feel that the center is a part of the hospital and that they are not losing their patients to it. Therefore, the center must be careful to provide clear and frequent communication with referring doctors. Follow-up should be done as much as possible within the hospital of origin of the patient and there must be active participation at all hospital conferences, ward rounds, etc. by the radiation oncology service.

The goals of such a conjoint center are to provide the patient with the treatment most likely to achieve cure or long-term control and palliation of the disease. This, of course, will change as new knowledge is gained. The conjoint radiation oncology center can help achieve this goal by making a broad base of professional consultation along with diverse and sophisticated equipment and techniques available to the patient. Research and training will be fostered in such a milieu. Perhaps, however, the most important advantage to be accrued from such a radiation oncology organization will be the impact on other areas of cancer management. It may provide the nucleus of similar organizations in medical oncology, surgery, and other specialties; thus, providing true interdisciplinary and coordinated cancer management within the general hospitals, currently the focus of our health care system. Multidisciplinary participation is important at all levels of management from the initial management decision to rehabilitation and follow-up. Such cooperative interhospital arrangements seem most conducive to providing such care in the setting of the general hospital while at the same time husbanding our resources and optimally using highly-skilled personnel and expensive, sophisticated equipment.

Author's address: Dr. SAMUEL HELLMAN, Department of Radiation Therapy, Harvard Medical School, 50 Binney St., *Boston, MA 02115* (USA)

Front. Radiation Ther. Onc., vol. 8, pp. 81–84
(Karger, Basel and University Park Press, Baltimore 1973)

The Triad of Responsibility in Cancer Care
Need for Further Definition

R. R. DEFFEBACH

Department of Radiotherapy, Peninsula Hospital and Medical Center, Burlingame, Calif.

The long-range goal in cancer management is total elimination of the disease process. From the current state of development it is more realistic to look at an intermediate goal, the reduction of mortality and morbidity to a minimum through ongoing basic research and the application of currently known treatment techniques. The purpose of my discussion today will be to provide suggestions and recommendations for achievement of this intermediate goal through the development of a mutuality of purpose among the government, university research and teaching programs and the community clinical cancer activities.

In this triad of responsibility for cancer, the government, the universities and community medicine, the analogy of the three-legged stool is convenient to consider. All three legs of the stool must be of equal length and must be directed towards a focal point, overall excellence of cancer services. The basic platform upon which this stool should rest is continual communication to collectively define areas of responsibility and means of solution, thus providing a firm, nontilted, nonbiased foundation for progress. Within this triad, each area of cancer concern must define its individual goals while always recognizing the definition of goals which is occurring within the other component parts. Government programs and funding, university teaching and clinical research programs, and existing patterns of practice in the community must all be dedicated to the primary concern, the individual patient.

If these basic principles are not recognized, we will be headed for a collision course of disparate goals. The National Cancer Institute is concerned that there must be an appropriate and responsible distribution of cancer monies made available to accomplish the mandates outlined by Congress and the President. Some centralization of planning and operational activities can seem from their vantage point to be the best means to achieve the solutions necessary. The university has the responsibility through teaching for maintenance of excellent care within the medical communities while furthering through basic and clinical research the techniques and knowledge of cancer disease processes. With this charge, it is natural to develop the position that even in the clinical management sphere all cases of difficulty or all cases subject to protocol evaluation should be treated at university centers. On the other hand, the communities feel that the primary physician is the most critical member of the medical team and that the logistical and social needs of the patient are of great importance, best satisfied by the most convenient and personal care possible. The communities also feel that with the increasing number of well trained oncologists, high-level services are available, capable not only of primary care, but also of effective cooperation in clinical research.

All three positions have considerable validity and all would seem to a certain degree to satisfy the basic goals, but there has been no consensus as to a proper balance of effort, thus resulting in independent decisions and positions, independently evolved. There must be agreement in assignment of responsibility.

The primary governmental responsibility should be catalytic and implementive rather than operational in nature. They have a national mandate to effect appropriate changes in many areas of medical care and they have been given large amounts of money to distribute in an effort to this. The development of cancer centers through governmental funding and peer review is a responsible way to assist this but it requires adequate input from the other two sectors of responsibility, the university and the community. The central evolution of a broad range of highly specific objectives arranged in shopping-list fashion with contract dispensation of specific activities takes away from the regions and communities the basic right of participation in the development of overall goals. For many there is the belief that regional and local input will provide better, more practical, more realistic solutions to the current problems since the mechanism is provided for adaptation to the regional variations, throughout the country, of degree of sophistication of cancer services.

The university teaching center has the primary responsibility for basic and clinical research and for the training of future physicians. The care of the individual patient, although obviously extremely important, and requiring the highest level of expertise possible, is a means to the end in accomplishing these goals, not a responsibility in itself. The development of the concept of cancer centers must not be looked upon by the universities as an opportunity to implement internal programs not previously funded, but an opportunity given by the government to work with the communities in the conceptual evolution of regional cancer care that will provide a proper balance of activity between research, teaching and improved clinical care while assisting the communities to improve their cancer services. Expansion of the clinical management sphere beyond the needs for teaching and basic and clinical research in most cases is not appropriate since the patient's needs clearly go beyond the area of treatment, relating also to his family, home, social and general medical needs.

The basic responsibility of the communities is to provide a high standard and high capability of clinical care for the cancer patient. Currently, 80–85% of the patients with cancer are being treated within the various communities in the nonteaching sphere, and the logistical, financial and social concerns of the patients would indicate that this continue. The universities are not capable and in most part do not desire to see a total expansion of clinical management through university center activities. Conversely, teaching and training is not the basic responsibility of the communities, but just as clinical management as a means to an end is a proper activity for the universities, training of medical people under university supervision can be a proper secondary activity of the communities.

The communities have in some cases over-reacted in an attempt to provide convenient and high-level care for its patients without adequate parameters to decide how these cancer service activities should be distributed. This has resulted in duplication, fragmentation and a cost-plus type of financing where the unit cost to patients have gone beyond acceptable levels. Volume of patient care, within certain limitations, results in both increase in professional level of care and decrease in unit cost of care. In spite of this, there has been a competitive and sometimes reactionary response on the part of institutions within communities to hold on to their patients. Fear on the part of communities of university or government disruption of practice patterns is in large part misplaced, but if there is not an adequate communication among the triad, the communities will feel disenfranchised and will make every effort to maintain and pursue their own course of action.

Assuming that all of the above is valid, it is apparent that considerable attention must be given to the development of mutually defined goals. This would hopefully provide a proper balance of activities among government, clinical and basic research workers, teachers and community medical representatives. It is suggested that inter-triad communication mechanisms be encouraged. Expansion of technical and advisory resources to aid this would be valuable in the design of acceptable, practical goals.

Regional cancer planning, recently encouraged by the National Cancer Institute, is potentially an important step. Regional planning must be done by people whose primary interest is cancer, but to establish credibility and to ensure implementation of planning suggestions, these councils must be chosen from as broad a base of interest groups and institutions within the region as possible. This implies counsel from existing intra- and inter-modality and inter-institutional organizations.

This is a complex and volatile task, and if professional and technical advisory resources were available, capable of expertise in a broad range of cancer problems, the taks of planning would be much easier. The development of regional agencies or foundations, cancer categorically oriented, would enable definition, in depth, of area needs, and assist regional councils in implementing solutions for defined needs. Such foundations could also generate local moral and financial support in areas where private funding would be appropriate.

Nonprofit foundation activity should also be encouraged to further define the proper balance of activity within the triad, perhaps acting as a national resource. An ongoing in-depth analysis of intermediate and long-range needs and goals is required to enable the collection of basic social and planning data related to the cancer problem. This would have particular relevance in the community sphere, where the large number of currently ill patients presents the largest and most complex organizational problems.

It is time to coordinate community medical effort in cancer with the government and with the teaching and research centers. Community-based, high-level clinical cancer facilities, requiring in almost all cases a consortium of institutions to satisfy professional and financial needs, can relate, at the same level of clinical excellence, to university-based regional cancer centers. However, all metropolitan hospitals cannot have cancer centers, and means to satisfy these conflicts must be evolved. Rural area needs must be recognized with considerable reliance placed upon support from centers.

Innovative thinking is required for all of these problems. Cancer should be primarily a concept, tailoring and molding existing regional professional and facilities resources, and providing a viable, continuous means of communication between basic and clinical research and the bedside of the patient.

Author's address: Dr. R. R. DEFFEBACH, Peninsula Hospital, 1783 El Camino Real, *Burlingame, Calif.* (USA)

Front. Radiation Ther. Onc., vol. 8, pp. 85–89
(Karger, Basel and University Park Press, Baltimore 1973)

Radiation Therapy in a Rural Setting

S. F. Thomas and C. K. Hubbard

Survey and Background

The justification for practicing radiation therapy in a rural setting is based on health needs of the population; not prestige or to have a complete medical center. Population density maps of the area shown the population distribution in relation to the medical personnel and facilities that are available (fig. 1, 2).

The population health needs and the cost of translocation must be supplied by the medical and lay community. The support of a tumor board, a tumor registry and an enthusiastic professional community are necessary

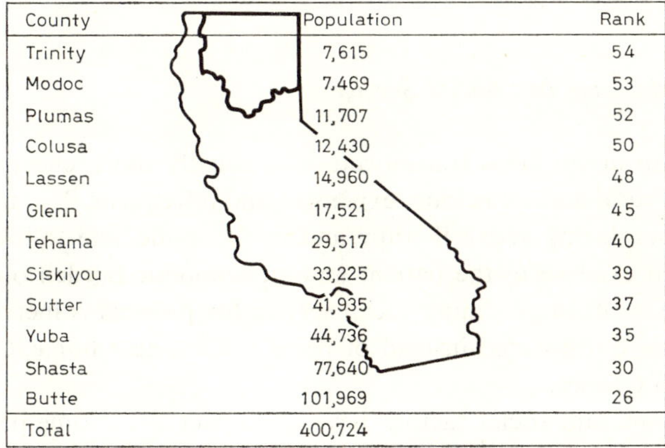

County	Population	Rank
Trinity	7,615	54
Modoc	7,469	53
Plumas	11,707	52
Colusa	12,430	50
Lassen	14,960	48
Glenn	17,521	45
Tehama	29,517	40
Siskiyou	33,225	39
Sutter	41,935	37
Yuba	44,736	35
Shasta	77,640	30
Butte	101,969	26
Total	400,724	

Fig. 1. Counties ranked by population among 58 Californian counties.

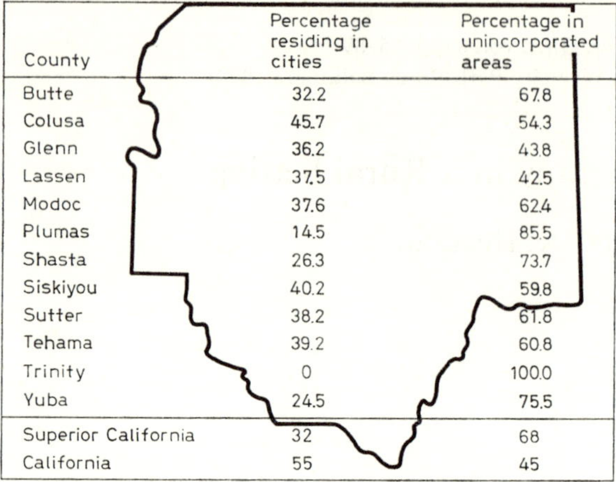

County	Percentage residing in cities	Percentage in unincorporated areas
Butte	32.2	67.8
Colusa	45.7	54.3
Glenn	36.2	43.8
Lassen	37.5	42.5
Modoc	37.6	62.4
Plumas	14.5	85.5
Shasta	26.3	73.7
Siskiyou	40.2	59.8
Sutter	38.2	61.8
Tehama	39.2	60.8
Trinity	0	100.0
Yuba	24.5	75.5
Superior California	32	68
California	55	45

Fig. 2. Percentage of population residing in cities or unincorporated areas by county.

features for success and self-instruction. No new treatment techniques or large series of patients will come out of a rural setting, but the rural practice can accommodate those patients which the urban center should not handle because of burgeoning numbers. For this reason there is a need for more rural radiation oncology centers. To become bogged down with size inefficiencies is not in the best interests of sound teaching. What are the efficient limits for carrying out radiation therapy? In the smaller centers 300 to 400 new patients a year are ample if there is proper technical and clinical backing.

Patient Translocation and Social Service

For patients in urban areas transportation is usually short, cheap and frequent; while in rural areas it is long, expensive and infrequent. The translocation of patients during active therapy and in the immediate follow-up period is an added expense to the patient and an economic burden on the community. Time spent in providing social service for patients is increased when the patient is translocated instead of being treated near home. Costs increase from 2 to 6 times.

The psychologic and social factors have an impact also. Some people would rather go elsewhere to get their treatment, but most are suited to their rural environment and do poorly when translocated for therapy.

Equipment

The rural setting needs better and more reliable equipment than an urban center. The advantage of the complex equipment may be offset by the inability to obtain proper engineering service without excessive cost. There is usually less money: available or potential.

Technical Help

Training of radiation therapy technologists usually takes in place urban centers and/or academic settings, both of which may offer advantages not found in the rural environment. Techincal help does not look to the rural community for employment. They must be either recruited to or educated in the rural setting; the latter being far more satisfactory for stability. Hopefully, as more physicians are trained in radiation oncology, more technicians and dosimetrists will become available to rural areas.

Radiological Physics

The backing of a physicist is needed not only to furnish machine calibrations, but to provide guidance in selection of treatment techniques. Complicated multiple field setups or irregular surfaces turn the consultation into a two-sided discussion. The telecopier and telephone make radiological physics services accessible. Computer-printed isodose distributions permit the weighing of alternatives. As these computer programs are refined, more of the physicist's time can be spent in improving the information put in the core of the machine and not spent on the day-to-day clinical problem solving.

Clinical Direction

Even with good technical help and radiological physics services, it is essential to have clinical direction. Discussion with super-peers of treatment policies or the treatment plan of the individual case is essential for education and maintenance of quality. With this type of clinical direction rural, radiation therapy is feasible. Not only are standards maintained by being helpfully watched, but the isolation of distance evaporates and the feeling of belonging to the radiation therapeutic community is realized.

Future

How to continue to meet the demands of population growth is a timely and pertinent question. The population growth in the next 25 years is projected to be 25% for this area, but the aging shift will almost double the numbers of patients. These estimates were made from 'Health plan for the 70's' published by the Superior California Health Planning Association (fig. 3, 4, table I).

Should present facilities be expanded or should a new geographic area be chosen and its facilities upgraded to accommodate the growth?

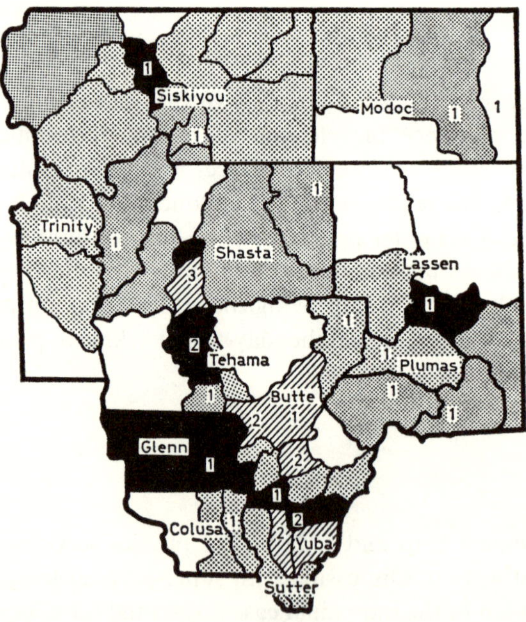

Fig. 3. Location and number of general hospitals.

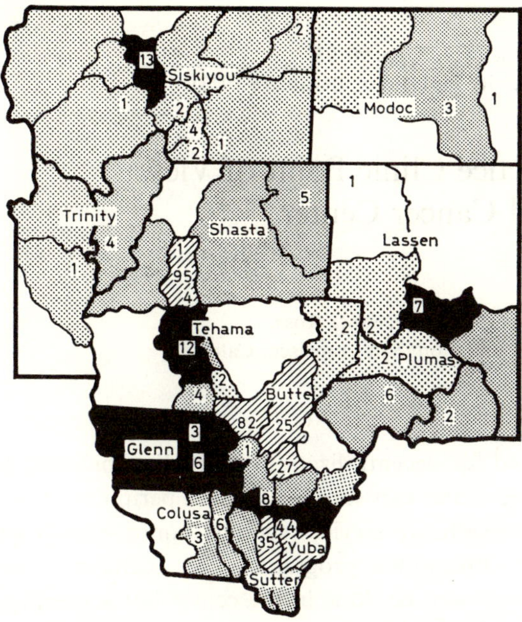

Fig.4. Location and number of physicians.

Table I. Population projections, 1975–2000

Area	1975	1980	1985	1990	1995	2000
Butte County	106,000	111,200	118,600	125,400	130,800	136,900
Colusa County	12,500	12,700	13,000	13,400	13,600	14,200
Glenn County	17,300	17,700	18,000	18,200	18,400	18,800
Lassen County	17,400	18,200	18,900	19,500	20,500	21,500
Modoc County	7,700	7,800	7,800	7,800	7,600	7,900
Plumas County	12,200	12,600	12,900	13,100	13,600	13,900
Shasta County	83,800	91,500	100,400	109,100	117,100	126,500
Siskiyou County	33,300	34,200	35,000	36,300	36,900	37,900
Sutter County	45,300	49,100	53,500	57,900	61,700	65,700
Tehama County	30,600	31,900	33,000	33,800	34,500	35,600
Trinity County	7,900	8,200	8,400	8,400	8,600	8,700
Yuba County	39,600	42,500	47,000	51,900	56,400	61,600

Author's address: Dr. S. F. THOMAS, Department of Radiation Therapy, N. T. Enloe Hospital, *Chico, CA 95926* (USA)

Front. Radiation Ther. Onc., vol. 8, pp. 90–93
(Karger, Basel and University Park Press, Baltimore 1973)

The Private Practice Clinic Point of View in the Integrated Cancer Center

A. F. SCHROEDER

Santa Rosa Radiation Therapy Center, Santa Rosa,
and West Coast Cancer Foundation, San Francisco, Calif.

There is a definite need for decentralization in the diagnosis and treatment of cancer. The cancer center can supply affiliated peripheral hospitals and private clinics with consultative services such as tumor boards, radiological physics and other educational programs. The treatment planning and radiation dosimetry may well be done in the center but screening procedures, diagnosis, surgery, radiation therapy and chemotherapy can be done in the peripheral center staffed by well trained personnel. This will require a multidisciplinary approach to all facets of the disease, particularly the cooperation and coordination of radiation therapy, surgery and chemotherapy. I feel that this can be achieved just as well in the local community as in a large major urban center. Success in cancer control in these communities depends on new discoveries in research, education, and the application of these discoveries to patient care. For this to be achieved, there must be good cooperation between the city and the periphery.

For many years it was thought that all patients with cancer had to be referred to the large major center for diagnosis and treatment. This has proved to be a social and financial hardship for many. There is a great cost to the patient, his family and the state or cancer society in bringing him to a city. This includes the medical cost, transportation, housing and food. The patient also will have to forego gainful employment which he may have been able to maintain if allowed to remain in his home town.

The sociopsychological aspects of uprooting the patient from his 'safe' environment and placing him in strange and often overwhelming new circumstances is not to be overlooked. The patient has suffered mental anguish over his disease but now has the added problems of loss of family, friends and familiar surroundings. This does not apply to all patients, but to many.

If these people could somehow be allowed to stay in their home communities with their friends, family and home surroundings, they could have a tremendous psychological boost, possibly continue to work at least part time and, above all, save the cost of additional housing, food and transportation. This goal would be on the premise that modern up-to-date equipment and services along with well trained radiation therapists and paramedical personnel are available in the home community.

With the aforementioned in mind, we designed and planned a new facility in Santa Rosa, California. This was accomplished with the aid of Enviro-Med, Inc. of La Jolla, California, a professional multidisciplinary planning firm. This firm carried on extensive research to determine whether a center such as this was needed in Santa Rosa, and what size facility was needed to care for the problems of the people. Approximately 3,000 ft^2 were allotted for the department. This was to include a reception area and waiting room, business office, two consultation offices, two examining rooms, bathrooms, a nurses' station, dressing areas, a work room, simulator-orthovoltage room, and a room for supervoltage equipment, in this instance a 4-MeV linear accelerator. This is located in a medical plaza with supporting services such as laboratory, pharmacy and diagnostic radiology readily available. There are also offices for all other types of medical specialties. The plaza is located in close proximity to four community hospitals, and numerous other private doctors' offices. It was designed to accomodate at least 50 patients per day under treatment, along with 10–15 follow-up examinations per day. We also considered having the capabilities of changes in type or number of treatment machines. It was our desire that the department have good functional design and also be pleasant and warm in appearance to the patients.

We anticipated a staff of two radiation therapists, two technicians, a nurse and an office manager. Physics to include treatment planning and dosimetry is coordinated through the city center with the aid of a xerox telecopier. The patient can be examined, contours made, sent to the city and plans returned in one day. Therefore, central planning and a computer can be utilized by many peripheral departments but are not necessary in each area. This results in a substantial savings in money and personnel. It still allows the small center to have the benefits of sophisticated dosimetry.

There is a close relationship between the local surgeons, internists, chemotherapists, pathologist, diagnostic radiologists and radiation therapist. Any clinician can present a patient to the bimonthly tumor board held at the various hospitals in the community and obtain recommendations for further diagnosis, therapy and follow-ups. Consultants for the major city centers actively participate in this program.

The center can enter patients into national protocol studies and participate in local, state and national data retrieval studies. This can allow cooperative studies to attain significant numbers of patients in shorter periods of time. If the staff is coordinated under one center and utilizes one group of physicists the techniques and dosimetry can be comparable.

The training of residents is of prime importance. There is a great variety of patients in the periphery that provide excellent material for teaching. There is also an opportunity for the resident in training to gain exposure to other than a large teaching center. There is the hope that this would ultimately lead to the placement of more well trained young radiotherapists in peripheral areas. There is a one-to-one relationship in teaching between staff and resident with the opportunity to see variable approaches to clinical problems by rotating through various departments. The resident can learn much about the financial functions of a private practice, something he cannot gain in a major center. Too often a trainee may later be assigned the task of starting a private department without any background or training in planning a department or in the field of economics.

Medical students need to learn about cancer, its diagnosis and treatment at an early point in their academic careers. The peripheral department can provide an opportunity for students who have received lectures in the major centers to go out and see surgery, radiation therapy and chemotherapy performed in the local communities. As many as 6 students at a time can rotate through the department and study the medical problem at the grass roots level. They can participate in the work-up and treatment of the patient and maintain a close staff-to-student teaching relationship. This is often not possible in a large center where the number of students is large and the number of staff teachers available small. The time to interest the student in cancer and encourage him to enter training in this field is during medical school. This may be an opportunity for our field to discover good new resident prospects.

The treatment of head and neck cancer requires good liaison with the fields of surgery, radiation therapy, chemotherapy and dentistry. We have rotated third- and fourth-year dental students through the department. It is advisable that the young dental student learn head and neck oncology not only in the classroom but in the field. This, too, can occur in the periphery. The rotation of these students has been well received both by the students and our staff.

There is a great need for well trained bright young technicians and dosimetrists in the field of radiation therapy. The centers in the city are attempting to train these people, but cannot provide enough staff and clinical material to train the numbers needed. We have joined the Santa Rosa Junior College and Santa Rosa Memorial Hospital in their technician training program. This requires regular didactic lectures, and on the job clinical training. The case material available provides another valuable part of their experience.

By treating patients with 4 fractions a week, there is time to go to the major center and participate in didactic lectures, laboratory and clinical research. The coordinated approach allows adequate well-trained personnel to cover each department and permit the staff and residents to attend national meetings and courses. Without this cooperation, time off would be at a premium.

I hope that as time passes more centers in the periphery can develop with the principals and goals that I have set forth, providing the needed care for the cancer patient in a peripheral area through cooperation with the major center in the city.

Author's address: Dr. ALAN F. SCHROEDER, Santa Rosa Radiation Therapy Center, Creekside Medical Plaza, 95 Montgomery Drive, Suite 118, *Santa Rosa, CA 95404* (USA)

Front. Radiation Ther. Onc., vol. 8, pp. 94–99
(Karger, Basel and University Park Press, Baltimore 1973)

The Cancer Center, the Community and Research

University of New Mexico Los Alamos Plan

M. KLIGERMAN

Institut

The Cancer Research and Treatment Center at the University of New Mexico, in Albuquerque, was planned by structural design and operational concept to provide modern cancer management for the people of this sparsely settled state. Interesting epidemiological observations are possible which could lead to the discovery of important genetic and immunological differences in a population which is composed of three cultural and ethnic groups, approximately 50% Anglo, 40% Spanish origin, and 7% Indian. There is also a black population accounting for 2%. Such differences, if uncovered, could be the key to defining the cause of certain cancers and thereby lead to new treatment methods.

Detailed records are maintained on the geographic location and type of cancer, the method of treatment and the place of treatment in the New Mexico Tumor Registry which is supervised by Dr. CHARLES KEY of the Medical Department of Pathology School. A second clinical investigative feature is the association with the π-meson human radiotherapy trials at the Los Alamos Scientific Laboratory. There will also be a laboratory research group in support of, and as a complement to, those whose clinical work raises new questions which require the laboratory for answers. However, basic investigation in tumor immunology, experimental oncology and radiation pathology are planned because of the interest and talent which exist at our university.

The clinical floor of the center (fig. 1) is planned for ease of rapid work-up and decision-making for the patient. The goal is to provide '1-day service' for the majority of the patients. In this day the patient will have an

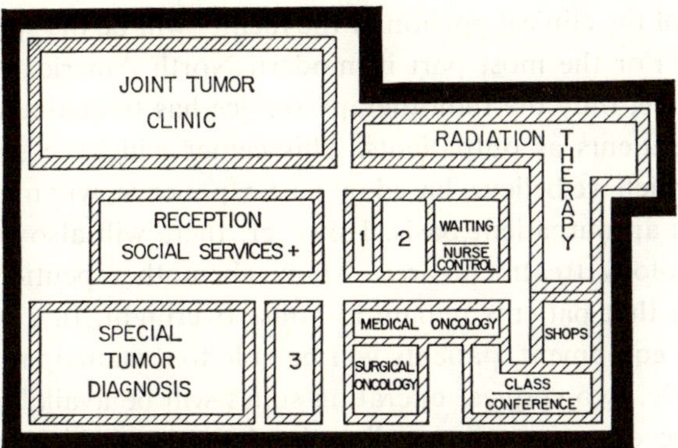

Fig. 1. Floor plan of the clinical area. The entrance is on the extreme left. The space is divided into those involved in the workup and follow-up of patients located to the left, and those specialized tumor therapy activities located to the right. 'Social services+' include in addition to representatives of the social service department, visiting nurse society representatives, clergy, dieticians, and transportation aids.
1 = laboratory medicine specimen collection sites
2 = offices for cancer trainees
3 = mold room, simulator room, and radiotherapy treatment planning

early-morning interview and examination by his responsible physician-oncologist and those trainees assigned to him. Diagnostic procedures such as those provided by diagnostic radiology, nuclear medicine and laboratory medicine will be ordered and obtained by suitable units within the center itself. There will be a collection of this data for the responsible physician in the early afternoon, and then presentation of all patients to the group of consultant oncologists later in the afternoon. To improve efficiency, a system of computer assignment of patients to specialized diagnostic equipment and collection of reports will be instituted.

In this way, every patient will be assured consultation with medical, radiation and surgical oncologists, specialty oncologists, and a pathologist who will be regularly assigned to the clinic with other members of the cancer center team. It is the intention to be in touch with the referring doctor before 17.00 h on the day of this exercise. This should decrease the number of anxious days the patient spends waiting for a decision. It will also reduce the patient's loss of income by shortening the number of days away from work required to reach this decision. It will provide for greater use of the patient's productive capacity as a worker in the community. Social service, dietitians, transportation aids, visiting nurses and Welfare Department representatives will have offices on the clinic floor.

A second feature of the clinical portion of the facility will be the specialized treatment center. For the most part in modern North American university oncology practice, only the radiotherapy service has treated a significant number of its patients as outpatients. This center will have such a radiotherapy facility which we believe, based on past experience, will manage 90% of its patients on an outpatient basis. However, there will also be included a medical oncology treatment area. Many chemotherapeutic procedures do not require that patients remain in-house overnight. In a 4-bed area, with appropriate equipment, patients will be able to remain up to 23 h as outpatients. Similarly, two surgical operating suites will be available for biopsies and other procedures including radium implantations which can be performed on an outpatient basis. Those patients who will remain at the medical center for treatment requiring hospitalization will be admitted to the appropriate existing service. A clinical research inpatient unit is planned, however, for research patients only.

Faculty appointments to the cancer research center will be dual ones. All members of the center will have appointments in the appropriate department of the School of Medicine corresponding to their specialty. It is believed that cancer research must have input from those developments in the basic science and clinical areas occurring outside the specific field of cancer investigation. This is the principal advantage a cancer research center – organized as a part of a general medical institution or medical center – has over isolated or freestanding cancer research institutes.

This center is to assist the referring doctor in managing his patient. Patients coming to the center without a family physician will not be turned away. However, with the patient's agreement, a doctor will be found for him in his local community. Three types of patients will be seen. Firstly, there are those sent by highly qualified specialists throughout the state who wish confirmation of their feeling about the patient or wish special studies performed which will be available at the center. Such patients after work-up will be referred back to this specialist. A second group will be patients referred by physicians who wish work-up and suggestions for management of a patient whom they suspect of having cancer but perhaps have not localized the tumor. Following decision, the referring physician in many instances would want the patient referred back to his community for his local specialist to manage. A third group will be patients sent by physicians asking for complete management of the patient at the center with referral back to the local physician at the conclusion of diagnosis and treatment.

All physicians in the state are invited to participate in this center. Those trained specialists in the community will be encouraged to give a regular portion of their weekly or monthly time to the center operation acting as the responsible physician. Other community physicians desiring postgraduate training will be accommodated either in blocks of time or on any regular weekly, fortnightly or monthly basis. These physicians will work-up patients for presentation to the responsible physicians and will, of course, participate in the new patient interdisciplinary conference in the afternoons.

Considerable thought has been given to methods of bringing modern cancer care to a sparsely settled population. New Mexico is the sixth largest state in the union areawise, but has a population of only 1,000,000 people. One-third of these resides in the Albuquerque area. It is planned to take teams of oncologists to outlying communities on a regular basis in cooperation with the county medical societies or appropriate hospital staffs. On the day the team of specialists spends with the local doctors, formal lectures will be given on subjects selected by the cancer center educational director and representatives of the community doctors. High point of the meeting, however, will be a working tumor conference in which the family doctor or responsible specialist of the community will present his patients to the visiting specialists in association with the rest of the doctors in his community. It will be a decision-making conference, not simply a teaching demonstration. Only through service to patients referred by the community doctors can rapport be established which will result in community doctors encouraging patients to participate in the clinical investigative programs of the center. The regular visits of physicians to the center as participants in its activities, and the regular visits of the team of oncologists to the outlyingcommunities will give the local doctor an opportunity to understand the research protocols, and to see them in operation. This author does not feel that significant numbers of patients will be sent centripetally to the center for clinical research unless centrifugal service to patients through their referring physician exists.

Though only in an early planning stage, a detection clinic will be developed at the center.

The Los Alamos Meson Physics Facility (LAMPF), directed by Dr. LOUIS ROSEN, is an open national facility. Through his efforts, outstanding support has been obtained from the Atomic Energy Commission and from the National Cancer Institute for the construction of a biomedical channel and a laboratory-clinic building. As in all other planned operations at, a users group advises Dr. ROSEN on the time alloted to projects for this channel. The radiotherapy subcommittee of the biomedical users group is currently chaired by Dr. MAX BOONE and has members from all over the country.

At the suggestion of Dr. PALMER SAUNDERS, Director, Division of Cancer Grants of the National Cancer Institute, the Committee for Radiation Therapy Studies has set up a subcommittee for human trials of pion radiotherapy. This is chaired by the author. This latter committee also counts among its membership persons from all over the country. A series of physical and biological experiments have been established by these committees which will be executed in preparation for human trials. An important feature of this activity will be the participation of scientists from all parts of this country and hopefully, from other nations, to be continued when human trials begin. These basic and clinical investigators will work for shorter or longer periods in conjunction with members of the Los Alamos Scientific Laboratory staff and the University of New Mexico faculty to complete first the preclinical programs in radiation biology and later the human trials.

The preclinical program will utilize cell culture techniques to look at the variation of relative biological effectiveness (RBE) with depth. Intestinal crypt cells and bone marrow will be studied as examples of cell renewal systems. Acute and long-time tolerance will be studied using skin, kidney, colon, spinal cord, heart and lung as representative systems. There will also be a program of experimental tumor therapy in mice and an attempt will be made to obtain spontaneous tumors in dogs for preclinical testing.

Human trials will begin with a phase I study to characterize normal and tumor tissue response. Multiple skin and pulmonary nodules will be test objects as well as large solitary lesions which are persistent or recurring. Following this 'clinical radiobiology', phase II studies will begin. The goal here will be the preparation for rapid and early clinical trials. Attempts will be made to establish preferred anatomic sites, to establish suitable dose schedules and to verify treatment planning. The committee has decided that phase II trials are to be the pilot studies for phase III and, therefore, all areas tested in phase II are potential candidates for phase III study. In the head and neck, the test areas will be gliomas of the brain (grades 3 and 4), all pyriform sinus lesions, advanced tonsil and anterior two-thirds of tongue lesions and T_3 and T_4 subglottic lesions. Transglottic lesions will also be studied. In the thorax, the esophagus, and superior sulcus tumors will be studied. The abdomen will contribute adult kidney carcinomas which are locally inoperable, the pancreas, the stomach, the rectum—clinically or surgically considered inoperable, the cervix of the uterus (stages 3 and 4), the bladder and the prostate. Soft tissue sarcomas and osteogenic sarcomas of the extremities are also considered good test sites.

In summary, a center devoted to clinical and laboratory investigation is planned which will combine efficient service to patients as a basis for improving cancer care in the State of New Mexico and as a method of obtaining a source of patients for research protocols. The center with its outreach program will attempt to be a model for similar operations in other sparsely settled states.

The extraordinary opportunity to study the radiobiology of negative π-mesons and eventually the human trials of cancer therapy with this charged particle at LAMPF will be unique in its operational plan which will utilize all available talent in the nation and hopefully from abroad to insure an intelligent and early answer to the value of such radiation in cancer management.

Author's address: Dr. M. KLIGERMAN, Cancer Research and Treatment Center, University of New Mexico, *Albuquerque, N M 87131* (USA)

Front. Radiation Ther. Onc., vol. 8, pp. 100–108
(Karger, Basel and University Park Press, Baltimore 1973)

A Program for a
Regional Radiation Therapy Network[1]

L. W. Brady, J. Mitchell and D. A. Lightfoot

Department of Radiation Therapy and Nuclear Medicine, Hahnemann Medical
College, Philadelphia, Pa., and Public Affairs Counseling, San Francisco, Calif.

Most data presented about radiation oncology or cancer center planning
relates to the 'models' that have been developed and that are appropriate to
necessarily unique circumstances and/or local situations. The purpose of the
present paper is to define a model that developed from unique conditions in
Philadelphia and its surrounding area. However, a second theme emerges that
can be directly related to other situations. The model of the Hahnemann
Regional Radiation Therapy Network is the *product* of long-term planning.
The process defines how we negotiated our way with 19 hospitals, each with
its own image, territory, sponsors, and alliances, old enmities and mistrusts,
to a viable, cooperating network of institutions bound together by common
interest and self-interest in a system of equals, formalized only by verbal
agreement and the trust which that represents.

Many impressive concepts and plans have foundered on the rocks of
institutional competitiveness and distrust. Indeed, many presentations in this
volume highlight just these problems. Yet few presentations offer guidance
on how cancer center planners should organize themselves to worry through
gaining the commitment and enthusiasm of all the legitimate interest groups
who must participate (because they have a great deal at stake) in the planning
of any workable center. This is true at the individual and departmental
level in a single institution, and true (but even more difficult) when dealing
with several institutions.

1   This project was supported by GDVRMP (project No. 20), by PHS Research Grant
No. 1-R10-CA-12252 from the National Cancer Institute, by PHS Research Grant No.
5-R10-CA-12478 from the National Cancer Institute, by the Friends of the Radiation Therapy Center, and by the Alperin Foundation.

An attempt will be made to present the historical development and also to offer guidelines that would be helpful in the development of such centers in other geographical areas.

Let us start by describing the situation as it existed at that time in Pennsylvania. It was our overall aim to make accessible to as many people as possible the best in modern cancer management and particularly radiation therapy. In the Greater Delaware Valley, 25,000 new cancer cases were estimated for 1969, of which about 12,000 would require radiation therapy for cure, palliation or as adjunct to surgery or chemotherapy. To serve these patients in optimal fashion required the orchestration of several institutions and the integration of the activities of a large number of diverse health professionals, each with special competence. It also required coordination in the use of sophisticated and often expensive equipment and facilities (each item of equipment costing in the range of $ 100,000–500,000). In the Philadelphia area, as in most places, only a few specialized centers possessed the needed range of resources. As a result, only a small fraction of patients could benefit from the increased cure rates and the improved and more effective palliation. Most of these resources were located in centers in Philadelphia. Patients were required to travel from their local area (distances of up to 100 mi) to be treated, or receive oftentimes less than optimal treatment utilizing local resources.

The cost of equipment and facilities and the relative scarcity of trained personnel had made past efforts tend to concentrate such expertise in one place, logically mostly around a medical school (almost inevitably in a large city). Yet, the initial management decision is the most critical component of the care of the patient with cancer. It was clear that for a variety of reasons large numbers of patients never reached, or benefited from, the concentration of expertise and resources in those cancer centers. We decided, therefore, to take that expertise into the local area, to reinforce their strengths and bolster their weakness. We started with a nongeographic functional definition of 'regional network', contacting those institutions with already existing linkages with Hahnemann.

In the initial discussions, it became immediately apparent that radiation oncologists and paramedical personnel in radiation therapy were in extremely short supply, making it difficult for practitioners not associated with the medical college to keep abreast of the new advances, not only in radiation therapy, but also in other techniques of cancer management. In general, the equipment necessary for proper radiation therapy was costly and, in many instances, was under-utilized in many of the participating institutions.

The initial discussions began among a group which included not only those physicians doing radiation therapy, but also pathologists, surgeons, cancer chemotherapists, gynecologists, etc. Out of these discussions came facts which were used in deriving the eventual system of cancer service delivery.

This was a central tenet of the negotiations, starting from where, based on a joint (ours and theirs) assessment of their strengths and weakness. We looked at the problems they faced as opportunities that the network could take advantage of and solve. In fact, several guiding principles proved essential to a cooperative and genuinely shared venture.

1. The development must start where the participants are.

2. All participants are equal (at least until *they* prove otherwise).

3. Everyone is explicitly assumed to have something to contribute. No one should be used to develop a list of names needed on the grant application.

4. Openness and honesty are key with no hidden agendas or gamesmanship.

5. No-one gets a free ride (the corollary to item 3 above). In the Hahnemann program everyone did his share and wrote his particular portion of the grant request.

6. No-one is locked into a single rôle or position. Mobility within the network was to be valued and encouraged.

These principles helped allay some of the interinstitutional jealousy, fears of dominance by the medical college and provided a means by which the regional network became in itself a focusing point within each of the institutions for their own resources, and a way of coming to grips with some of their own internal problems.

The network of coordinated institutions provided us with access to the initial cancer management decision, a decision most often made in a physician's office, the general medical clinic, the community hospital or other sites of primary medical care. In order that the integration of specialized radiation therapy management within the overall system of health care could be achieved, the following goals in cancer management necessary to increase curability and improve palliation were postulated by the planning group:

1. The organizational structure for cancer management should provide for only a single optimal level of care.

2. This optimal management should be available to all, regardless of economic, social or geographic considerations.

3. Multidisciplinary participation in prevention, diagnosis, treatment and follow-up must be available in any circumstance in which cancer management is undertaken.

4. Currently limited highly trained personnel, sophisticated equipment and facilities for radiation therapy must be efficiently utilized with attention to minimizing the cost consistent with high-quality care.

5. Sufficient numbers of highly qualified personnel in all of the cancer-related disciplines must be trained.

6. Maximum information must be derived from all patients with cancer as a basis for study of the disease and its treatment.

7. Recent advances must be rapidly translated into clinical application.

In order to accomplish these stated goals, we needed to redefine the traditional concept of a cancer center. In the past, this has meant a physical structure, housing many cancer-related activities. Frequently, arrangements were made with other institutions for consultation and patient referral in a *center satellite* relationship.

This concept was defined in the 1968 report of the Committee for Radiation Therapy Studies, 'A prospect for radiation therapy in the United States', in which three types of facilities were detailed. Implicit in this stratification were three levels of patient care. The level of care was, therefore, often determined by the patient's point of entry into the system which, in turn, depended upon geographic or economic considerations, patterns of referral, customs or accident.

The planning group wrestled with how to operationalize its previously stated goals in a different way. After much discussion and argument, it came up with a definition of a 'network'. It redefined the center concept as a broad functional entity, embracing all the cancer-related activities of the 19 co-operating institutions and professional individuals. The main characteristics were: availability of specialized care at the primary management site, common utilization of personnel and equipment, a single system of records, and assurance of equality of care regardless of the point of entry.

Thus, the concept proposed was not one of the *center* of a whole circle of activities, but rather *it was the circle* itself. An advantage of this concept was that, through close collaborative arrangements, in time the data base for clinical research could be enlarged to include essentially all patients with cancer. This is possible and it leads eventually to collaborative arrangements insuring qualified professional evaluation, compatible records, uniform treatment policies, cooperative clinical investigation, careful and complete follow-up and close communication and interaction among involved professional personnel. In this manner a rapid transfer of research advances into clinical practice is made possible. This milieu also offered an ideal environment for training in any of the cancer-related disciplines by giving extensive experience in a particular discipline while heightening awareness of the important rôles of related disciplines.

It was in this form that a grant application for partial support of such a concept was written and submitted to the Greater Delaware Valley Regional Medical Program. The main objectives were described as:

1. To explore as a pilot study the potentials for the delivery of comprehensive oncologic services to any system of a medical school and its cooperating hospitals.

2. To explore the feasibility of including other medical schools and their cooperating hospitals in a broad partnership for the delivery of oncologic service on a regional basis.

3. To explore new and innovative concepts in terms of education and training.

This grant was, after considerable delay, funded. The program, as it currently operates, integrates the radiation therapy facilities at 8 major institutions (Reading Hospital, Crozer-Chester Medical Center, St. Joseph's Hospital, Pennsylvania Hospital, Lankenau Hospital, Allentown Hospital, Harrisburg Polyclinic Hospital and Monmouth Medical Center) with a number of smaller institutions, with plans to add others later (fig. 1).

Physics and dosimetry activities are proceeding in three stages: the standardization of all supervoltage and megavoltage quality machines as to output and data needed to compute isodose data *for each machine;* establishment of a computer and treatment planning system; and *invivo* and phantom verification of delivered dosage.

In accordance with our basic philosophy, the participants of the 8 major institutions have acquired their own full-time radiation therapy coverage, as well as full- or part-time physics coverage.

As previously mentioned, the program is partially supported in its present, demonstration phase by the Greater Delaware Valley Regional Medical Program. However, its major service aspects should permit self-supporting operation on a fee-for-service basis as the program benefits become apparent to the medical community and the public generally.

Our experience shows that proper organization and function of the participants are essential for success. After considerable discussion with the participants and with others who had dealt with similar questions, we decided to base our plan for organization and management on 4 key prin-

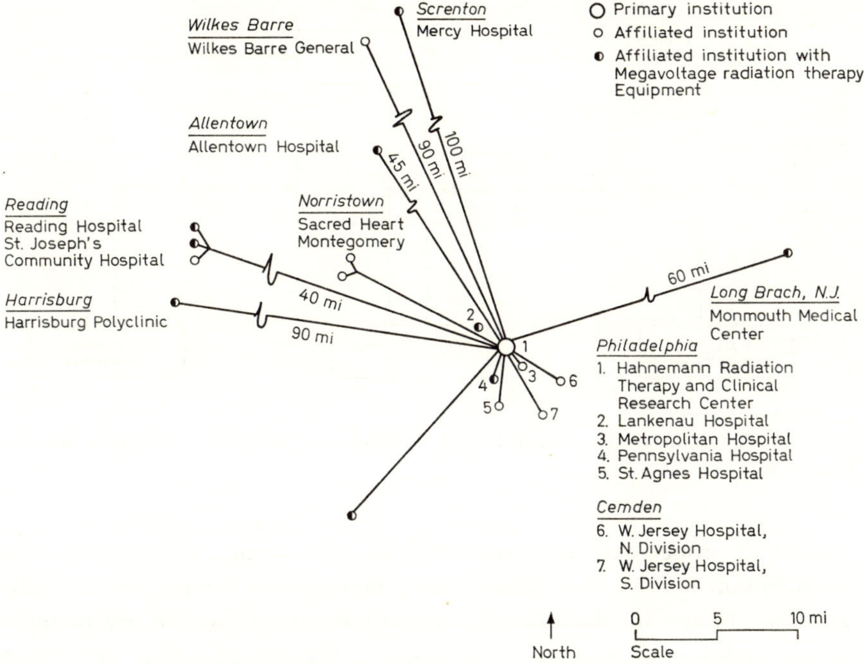

Fig. 1. Regional radiation therapy network.

ciples: (1) management within a *democratic* framework; (2) treatment of patients as *close to home* as medically feasible; (3) *extensive service* to the network by the medical school center, and (4) *feedback* from the participating hospitals.

1. *Management.* Although the medical school center was the natural activity focus, parity was essential among all participating physicians and institutions, with full representation and voice in the administrative board (fig. 2). Agreements were often verbal rather than formal, since they were based on mutual interest in solving a common problem. A strong effort was made to involve all cancer-relevant departments, not only radiation oncology, but surgery, gynecology, internal medicine, hematology, pathology, etc. Clinical faculty appointments were encouraged where significant participation was involved, to emphasize the cooperative nature of the program.

2. *Local treatment where feasible.* It is neither possible nor desirable to treat all patients at the major center. However, several prerequisites are

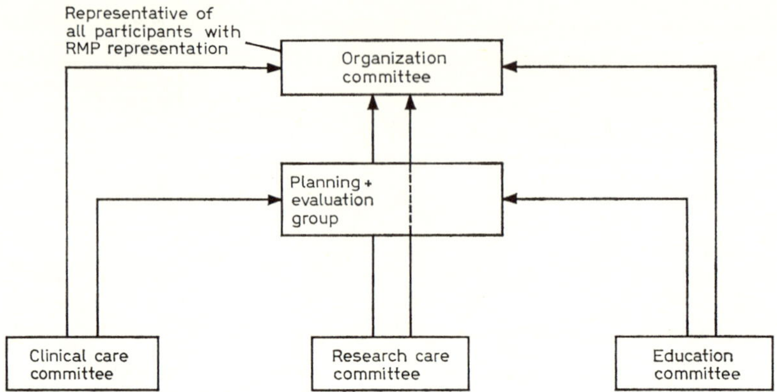

Fig. 2. Administrative structure for Hahnemann Regional Radiation Therapy Network.

needed to properly treat the majority near their homes. Firstly, there must be optimum utilization of supervoltage machines in the region. Secondly, accurate dosage standardization, calculation and evaluation are required. Finally, additional personnel and in-service training as well as new equipment and accessories are essential to meet the need for definitive therapy and increased patient load.

3. *Extensive service by medical school center.* Patient service falls into three categories. Professional and technical paramedical help is needed for physics, dosimetry and treatment planning. This was provided both remotely by means of telemetry and computer techniques, as well as through on-site visits for dose standardization, verification, and other functions. Clinical consultation is provided both remotely by telemetry and telephone and in person by visiting specialists at tumor clinics in participating hospitals as well as in reciprocal visits to the center. Finally, the major medical school center increasingly tends to deal with more difficult treatment problems. At present, these include those requiring specialized shielding techniques (as in Hodgkin's disease and seminoma), hyperbaric oxygen therapy in combination with radiation therapy, and electron beam and high (LET) radiation equipment.

The medical school center actively participates in training physicians as well as radiation physicists, biologists and technologists, both at the center and at participating institutions. This is in addition to continuing medical education programs and ready consultation regarding specific patients.

Research must proceed in two parallel directions. The first leads to improvement in radiation therapy including both dosage evaluation and equipment and accessory design. The second leads to ongoing biological research to develop more effective ways to treat cancer. Such work is carried out in the radiation biology laboratories and medical school generally, and on a clinical level at all hospitals in the administrative center.

4. *Feedback from participating hospitals.* To best serve the patient, the system must provide for a free flow of information. All physicians have much to learn from each others' experiences, both formally in a tumor registry and on a person-to-person basis in patient consultation and follow-up. In addition, an extensive regional program can provide both the variety and numbers of disease for participation in significant clinical trials, which are essential to provide a sound basis for medical advances. The Hahnemann Regional Radiation Therapy Network now treats 3,100 new cases of cancer per year (1972) using radiation therapy techniques.

Feedback and joint evaluation of both clinical and management data is crucial to long-term planning and development of the network. For, in truth, the planning process is iterative, never-ending, with modification of form and content required to minimize the inevitable *lag* between the capacity and organization of the network to respond to *its perception* of the problems of the area that it should solve, and the real nature of the problems as they actually exist. Organizations seldom take their final form from a single act of design. They grow into their identities. Their evolution depends upon a rigorous selection from all the characteristics of their prospective constituencies or 'clientele' from activities and situations that by their nature can never be fully enumerated. If this process is to be consonant with the *realities* of the local area, feedback and evaluation are critical.

Summary

The Hahnemann Regional Radiation Therapy Network Program has evolved from both interinstitutional cooperation and extensive conferences over a period of several years. It is designed to provide organizational, professional and technical means for improved radiation therapy for cancer patients in the Delaware Valley. It is now operating as a pilot program, which emphasizes flexibility and cooperation, and which may serve as a prototype for similar programs adapted to meet the diverse medical needs of our state.

Even though the regional program centered around the Hahnemann Medical College has been under way and funded for only 18 months, there are significant evidences that a major impact has been made, not only upon the clinical practice relating to radiation therapy and cancer, but also on the teaching and education within the region.

Responsibility of the system for the quality of all components and disciplines must be shared by all the participants. It is no longer acceptable to be content with achieving high quality only within a narrow discipline or institutional confine. The advantages of closeness to primary care, previously the province of the private physician in community hospital, combined with a demonstrated excellence of the specialized cancer management facility can be achieved through this unique regional arrangement.

Author's address: Dr. LUTHER W. BRADY, Department of Radiation Therapy and Nuclear Medicine, 230 North Broad Street, *Philadelphia, PA 19102* (USA)

Front. Radiation Ther. Onc., vol. 8, pp. 109–119
(Karger, Basel and University Park Press, Baltimore 1973)

Social Work in the Cancer Center

PATRICIA FOBAIR

Zellerbach Saroni Tumor Institute, Mount Zion Hospital and Medical Center,
San Francisco, Calif.

Introduction

Social work is ideally an important humanizing influence felt throughout the cancer center. The social worker is a valuable member of a circle of specialists and acts on behalf of the cancer patient *and* the physician. The radiotherapy department of the cancer center offers the social worker an environment with maximum opportunity to help the patient. Here follows a history that illustrates these statements.

In August, 1971, 6-year-old Billy traveled with his young parents to the radiotherapy department for treatment. The youngster had been referred by a physician in a neighboring area, where the family had a new home.

Billy's diagnosis was Wilm's tumor, grade IV. The treatment regime was to include preoperative radiation therapy to be followed by surgery, postoperative radiation therapy, and later chemotherapy (actinomycin-D). The initial treatment course would require 6 weeks.

The radiotherapist brought the parents to meet me shortly after their initial interview: This was the problem: the physicians were certain that the child must have therapy in the center, but the parents felt it would be impossible to bring Billy to San Francisco for treatment while trying to cope with numerous other problems that faced them.

Billy's father, a proud, headstrong man, was hoping to enroll in a new state college, a step that would fulfill his dream of earning a degree and, through his college training, make life better for his family. A Navy veteran, he had managed to complete 2 years of junior college by going to classes at night and supplementing his G. I. Bill allowance by moving furniture during the day.

The family was in the process of settling down in their newly-rented home when Billy began to show symptoms of his disease. Now transportation problems sprouted painful conflicts for the parents, the father, not only reluctant to give up any part of his plans for attending school, also needed the family car to commute. Billy was not an only child. There was a 3-month-old baby girl who also needed much of the mother's attention.

Financially, the situation was threatening. The family was living on the father's final pay check from the job he had given up before their recent transfer. Eager to move, the parents had rather unrealistically, but hopefully, counted on the G. I. Bill allowance to arrive early, a phenomenon that had never before occurred. Both parents wondered how the 90 mi day commute to San Francisco would be possible.

There was no point in focusing on the parent's reluctance to meet Billy's need for treatment. When they finished explaining their difficulties, the social worker asked the father if he would consider transfering from the more distant school to the state college in San Francisco. Would they consider moving into the area, closer to the treatment facility? The social worker reasoned that it would be months before Billy's need for therapy was finished. The parents agreed to try.

San Francisco State College accepted the late transfer 'due to the medical emergency in the family'. The family moved closer to the hospital. Medical expenses and emergency funds were arranged through the welfare department. The father's back injury led to a referral to the State Vocational Rehabilitation Program which was able to supplement his G. I. Bill allowance to meet his school expenses.

Today, some 13 months later, Billy has completed therapy and has remained well. His father has finished his third college year with honor roll grades. Billy's mother was able to take care of both of her children without unsual difficulty during Billy's therapy.

The psychological problems that Billy and his parents experienced were held at a minimum by stabilizing the homelife.

While social work can be helpful to patients, there is an interplay of factors which affect the success of a social services program. Such variables include the social worker's ability, the cancer patients' need and willingness to accept help, and interdepartmental communication problems.

I want to discuss these factors and propose some thoughts for the new cancer center.

Social Work in the Cancer Center; a Definition and Description

Social work in the cancer center is the process of defining patients' problems and providing the services and counseling that facilitates patients' medical care. The social worker helps patients cope with or tolerate the treatment program, mobilizes and supports their will to live, and helps some patients plan for their lives when therapy is completed, i. e. rehabilitation. For other patients, the social worker becomes the friend who will stand by them when they die.

The social worker can often bridge a communication gap between the patient and the physician. She can facilitate the smooth flow of patients into the treatment program by solving the problems which prevent patients from keeping appointments. Also, by developing good relationships with urban and rural community agencies, she helps create a positive feeling towards the cancer hospital in the minds of the public.

How does she do it? What is the social worker's method? The social worker listens to the patients' problems, anticipates solutions that may help, and facilitates the patients' ability to help themselves. She relates with patients, their families and community agencies. She understands that some patients need to maintain rigid control over their destiny, while other patients will respond by dependent or regressive behavior. Some patients, experiencing an acute sense of, 'threatened loss,' actively fear any separation from family and friends. The social worker understands the patients' defensive behavior as a demonstration of their need to maintain psychological equilibrium as they cope with new realities of their situation.[6]

In the developing cancer center concept, the relationship between the social worker and the outlying community is of great importance. In communities distant from the cancer hospital, patients and agency personnel may be initially fearful or suspicious of the urban hospital. Resistance to treatment may develop because patients do not want to leave home for 6–8 weeks, or when physicians and agency personnel fail to anticipate the needs of the patient who travels to the urban center.

Sometimes it takes the dramatic example to convince the reluctant agency to improve procedures. In one Northern California community, the writer labored continuously to develop better referral planning with doctors and agency personnel. Yet, one day an elderly man arrived from this community more dead than alive! Discharged from his local hospital the day before, he had barely endured the ten-hour drive to the City, hastily arranged for him by his friends in the Sheriff's Department. Though sent to us for a six week course of radiation therapy for cancer of the larynx, he had arrived without x-rays, slides, or other medical records, nor had any financial arrangements been made for his stay. While the physicians and staff were busy getting the patient examined and admitted into the hospital, I called the agencies involved to see what had gone wrong. Everyone thought that someone else was helping the patient! Using this example as ammunition within their departments, both the local welfare department and the American Cancer Society unit reorganized their procedures to expedite the journey of future patients. We have all experienced better continuity of care since then.

Working with cancer patients in a group is another method which has stimulated my thinking. During recent years, there have been social work efforts with groups at the University of California Hospital, Stanford Medical Center, and many other institutions. The social work staff at Memorial Hospital in New York has worked with groups of patients and their relatives in both the pediatric and rehabilitation units [11]. In February, 1972, I formed a group with patients and staff in our radiation therapy department. The group was formed because it was observed that many patients seem to lose direction when therapy was completed. They became more depressed and there was evidently an unmet need. Called a staff-patient discussion group, we have been meeting weekly for 1½ hours per session. Patients are invited, but not urged to attend. Those who do choose to come once, or more often, seem to have several characteristics:

(1) they do not totally deny their anxiety or depression over their illness and treatment program; (2) they are willing to talk with their peers and the staff members about their disease and are not afraid to tell their story, and (3) they seem to need contact with others outside their families where it may be safer to confide their troubles. There are 10 regular patient participants and 3 or 4 staff, including one or more radiotherapy residents.

Discussions cover difficulties patients have faced since learning their diagnosis. The greatest need for many patients is to verbalize repeatedly the story of their most difficult moments [5]. Fears about death are mentioned but do not seem to dominate discussion. More important are discussions of the problems inherent in living with cancer, such as losing ones job, sleeplessness, loss of energy, the need for readjustments in one is life. Some patients discuss with the residents their fantasies about cancer development in the body and use the opportunity to register complaints about the treatment program.

All patients who attend seem to benefit from the realization that they are not the only ones who feel 'victimized'. Many express relief in discovering that they are not as ill as they might be. A psychiatrist patient once commented that the worst thing about having cancer was the feeling of 'inferiority' that it gave him regarding his body. Group participation seems to elevate the members' feelings towards themselves.

We have noticed that several patients who have participated for 3 or 4 months have experienced a kind of psychological rehabilitation. For example one 63-year-old lady was initially very angry with her physician and her former employer. Her illness had left her handicapped in body movement and she had lost her position, held for 25 years. Now, several months later, having relied on the group members for support, she is no longer angry and has found herself a volunteer position where her talents as a medical secretary are appreciated. She has renewed confidence in herself. Another patient, a retired businessman and amateur golfer, denied his depression initially but refused to return to golf. His wife was concerned that he was preoccupied with symptoms and was overprotecting himself. He had lost confidence in himself. He is now using the group to mobilize himself psychologically and to enjoy the remaining years of his life. Many other patients seem less depressed and are generally more active. A side-effect of the group is the new sense of intimacy that staff and patients feel for one another. The patients, as the consumers of treatment, give staff feedback regarding the depersonalizing aspects of their treatment programs.

What Problems Does the Social Worker Face in the Delivery of Service to Various Medical Sections of the Cancer Hospital?

While social work assistance should be available to patients throughout the cancer hospital, the social worker encounters the patient in a medical environment that changes as the patient moves from the diagnostic or surgical section to the radiotherapy and chemotherapy sections. Not only is there a great deal of medical care which keeps the cancer patient bouncing back and forth among medical units [10], the quality of doctor-patient communication appears to change from one service to the next.

For example, during diagnosis and surgery, the physician may withhold from a patient medical information concerning his case. He has a delicate communication problem. He wants the patient's cooperation with procedures but he hopes to avoid his excessive anxiety. The doctor may wait to talk frankly with the patient about the diagnosis until he has something positive to say. The patient, on the other hand, may wish to deny any possibility of serious disease [3], or he may indicate an eagerness to hear the truth [1]. At one hospital it was found that the majority of cancer patients whose disease was regarded as curable were told about their malignancy, while those patients with inoperable conditions reported receiving more varied information from physicians, including in some instances an avoidance of any discussion of diagnosis [9].

Such a variety of doctor-patient communication presents a number of problems to the social worker in her work with the patient. While she can be of help in providing supportive services to the patient, she may lose a valuable opportunity to talk more frankly.

Studies at Memorial Hospital in New York have shown that women who exhibited normal concern and mild depression in anticipation of a hysterectomy, but accepted the operation for the expected relief of symptoms and return to health, had minimal to moderate psychological difficulties postoperatively; while patients who showed little or no anxiety beforehand had the greatest difficulties afterwards [2]. A frank discussion between the presurgical patient and the social worker could be helpful to the surgeon in providing emotional support for those patients who are anxious and depressed, and in determining which patients might become most depressed after surgery.

The radiotherapy department presents many advantages for a more cooperative effort between physicians and social workers. The physician may have a communication advantage in the radiation therapy department. Since the patients' diagnostic work-up is usually completed before the referral, the radiation therapist can begin his relationship with the patient with a discussion of diagnosis and need for therapy.

Open communication between the staff and patients can be achieved in the radiation therapy department where physicians are present during the working day, members of the staff have access to each other and informal discussion about patients' needs is possible. Many patients are ambulatory outpatients and come for therapy over a long period of time. They are able to see their physician more often and in a less formal atmosphere than the usual doctor's office. All these factors enhance communication.

The social worker naturally benefits from the physician's availability and frankness with the patient. She finds that patients are less apt to deny negative feelings and more ready to discuss their problems. The length of treatment time enhances her ability to 'get to know' the patient.

Social work with patients undergoing chemotherapy is less straight-forward. As an auxillary to the physician, I have found the patients' communication with me more guarded. Here I have the problem of knowing how much to say and what question to ask. With what delicacy or intrusiveness should I talk to the patient? ABRAMS[1] pointed out that patients who were formerly direct about their medical situation became amnesiac about the course of illness, focused on bodily symptoms or even suggested other possible pathologic processes.

Even with patients I have known well for months, I find that the patients' ability to utilize social services changes during terminal care. While some patients are afraid of losing contact with reality, their friends and relatives, others appear to withdraw from people at this point [1]. Their increasing dependency on everyone around them may require a 'mothering' style of emotional support. All of these factors influence the social worker's ability to help the terminal patient.

Which Cancer Patients Need Social Sercives and which Cancer Patients Will Use the Social Services Offered?

Most of the current medical literature is directed towards describing fatally ill cancer patients and their need for better care from physicians, nurses and social workers [8, 9]. More work is needed to describe the needs of patients who survive. Although work has been done to enumerate problems, no effort has been made to describe which patients used the services offered. In one study, 700 instances of problems were tabulated from in-depth interviews with 60 fatally ill patients [8]. The problems included difficulties in family relationship and changes in mood.

It would seem that there is a gap between the observable needs and the patients' actual use of services. In a study sponsored by the American Cancer Society in 1969, we interviewed 134 patients in the radiation therapy department at Mount Zion Hospital [4]. This group represented the new patient load for a 2-month period. The point of the study was to gather basic data from the patients; to have medical and technical staff rate them for diagnosis, prognosis and ability to cope with the treatment program, and to observe which patients used social services and which did not, noting the service needs requested and given.

The results of the study showed that 51% of the patients used social services for a variety of reasons. Initially, 60% of the 68 patients who used social services were referred for help with tangible needs, i. e. transportation, financial assistance and housing. 40% were referred for emotional support during therapy and assistance in solving personal or family problems.

At the end of the study, 60% of the patients were visiting the social worker for emotional support, 35% were utilizing help in solving problems, 57% received help with transportation, 37% with financial assistance, and 28% received help in locating housing, nursing homes or housekeepers.

Only one significant difference could be found between patients who used services and those who did not. This had to do with the patients' attitude towards talking with a social worker. Those patients who rated themselves with a 'positive attitude' also used social service 82% of the time, while those patients with a less positive or negative attitude used services less often. Other factors, possibly related to the patients' use of services, included sex (women used social services more than men), living alone, having a low income and, not surprisingly, patients who were rated by their physicians as having a poor prognosis.

It is my belief that more than 51% of the patients had needs which could be tabulated, but their willingness to use the services available was contingent upon factors and attitudes only partially anticipated in the study.

What Kind of Social Work Program Would Best Assist the Patient in the Cancer Center?

If we define the cancer center beyond the hospital and look upon a whole community or region as a cancer center, three points come to mind that would shape the social work program.

1. The patient-social worker contact should begin in the patient's home community be continued during hospital care flowing back to the home community for follow-up.

2. The medical, social work and patient-care programs should be so well integrated in the cancer hospital that teamwork and communication would be maximized and patient's transfers throughout the hospital would be kept at a minimum.

3. To meet the needs of the cancer center staff, an ongoing training program for hospital and community service personnel should be established in oncology, psychiatry and social work.

Social concern for the cancer patient should begin in the patient's home community. The American Cancer Society staff could, with referral from physicians, act as initiators of services to patients at home and provide co-ordination of local community services with the cancer hospital before the patient's arrival.

While social service should be available throughout the hospital, an integrated approach is needed among medical, nursing and social work programs which will allow better teamwork and communication among staff members [10]. Such a program would not only discourage multiple patient transfers to various medical units, it would discourage the unnecessary psychological regression among the patients. One report from an east coast hospital describes the creation of an antiregressive atmosphere on a medical oncology service. The program began with a psychiatrist consulting with the nursing staff once a week. Thereby meeting some of the nurses needs for ventilation and exploration of their feelings. It developed as the nurses began spending more time talking with the patients in their rooms. Subsequently the stronger patients began to assume some of the nursing tasks such as filling water bottles, making beds for themselves and sicker patients, answering telephones and running errands. The 'revolution' reached the point where the nurses were able to have each newly admitted patient oriented to the ward by a welcoming group of older patients [7]. Eventually, a communal patients' dining room was established which allowed lonely and isolated patients to talk to each other. The patients discovered new psychological strength that came from their shared experiences. Programs like this one should be encouraged in cancer centers.

A new cancer center concept involving coordinated patient care and an integrated hospital care system suggest a need for the old staff to learn new skills. Community service people need to learn more about the disease and its treatment while medical staff members need to enlarge their perception of the patients' psychological experience. Using both the local community and cancer hospital as teaching centers, programs can be developed to meet these needs.

Research Possibilities

There are several research possibilities which might lead to collaborative efforts between physicians, social workers and other staff.

1. A more discriminating study is needed relating the medical and emotional needs of cancer patients, describing their ability to use the help of staff during different periods of their disease.

2. Related to this, there are studies to be done in the area of the stress-distress syndrome. Does stress in life necessarily lead to distress emotionally or physically? Some interesting work with cancer patients during the diagnostic period has been done [10].

3. Why not study cancer patient survival from emotional and psychological viewpoints as well as by treatment modalities? What are the rehabilitation needs of the cancer patient who survives?

4. Better medical-social research is needed to study the relationship between chronic depression and physical illness. What is the rôle of emotional factors in stimulating disease among cancer patients?

To summarize, while social work services can be an important part of cancer center, adding much to the patient care program, there is an interplay of factors which affects the success of the program. The social worker's success will be partially dependent upon her ability, the patient's acceptance and willingness to use social service, and the atmosphere and communication of the medical service, even the overall patient care program of a cancer center. The physician, as leader of the team, can lend his support to better patient care in the cancer center, thereby facilitating a more successful program.

References

1 ABRAMS, R. D.: The patient with cancer. His changing pattern of communication. New Engl. J. Med. *274:* 317-322 (1966).

2 DRELLICH, M. G., BIEBER, I., and SUTHERLAND, A. M.: The psychological impact of cancer and cancer surgery VI. Adaption to hysterectomy. Paper presented at the 9th Annual Cancer Symp. of the James Ewing Society. Cancer *9:*1120-1126 (1956).

3 EASSON, W. M.: Care of the young patient who is dying. J. amer. med. Ass. *205:* 203-207 (1968).

4 FOBAIR, P. A.: Mount Zion patient service demonstration project. A final report. Unpublished mimeograph (American Cancer Society, Washington 1970).

5 HOROWITZ, M. J. and BECKER, S. S.: The compulsion to repeat trauma. J. nerv. ment. Dis. *153:*32-40 (1971).

6 KATZ, J. L.; WEINER, H.; GALLAGHER, T. F. and HELLMAN, L. Stress, distress, and ego defenses. Arch. gen. Psychiat. *23:*131-142 (1970).

7 KLAGSBRUN, S. C.: Cancer, emotions, and nurses. Amer. J. Psychiat. *126:*71-78 (1970).

8 KOENIG, R. R.: Fatal illness. A survey of social service needs. Social Work *13:*85-90 (1968).

9 PAYNE, E. C. and KRANT, M. J.: The psychosocial aspect of advanced cancer. J. amer. med. Ass. *210:*1238-1242 (1969).

10   SHELDON, A.; RYSER. C. P., and KRANT, M. J.: An integrated family oriented cancer
     care program. The report of a pilot project in the socio-emotional management of
     chronic disease. J. chron. dis. *22:*743-755 (1970).
11   TRACHTENBERG, J. M.: Team Involvement and the Problems Incurred. Unpublished
     paper presented at 15th Annual Clinical Conference on Progress in the Rehabilitation
     of the Cancer Patient. M. D. Anderson Hospital, Houston, Texas, 1970.

Author's address: Miss PATRICIA FOBAIR, M. S. W., Claire Zellerbach Saroni Tumor
Institute, Mount Zion Hospital and Medical Center, P. O. Box 7921 *San Francisco,
CA 94120* (USA)

Front. Radiation Ther. Onc., vol. 8, pp. 120–125
(Karger, Basel and University Park Press, Baltimore 1973)

Radiological Physics in a Cancer Center and Other Comments

R. J. SHALEK

Physics Department, The University of Texas at Houston, M. D. Anderson Hospital and Tumor Institute, Houston, Tex.

Introduction

During the past 4 years I have had the opportunity to be associated with two cooperative programs in radiological physics related to radiation therapy. The Radiological Physics Center, initiated by the Committee for Radiation Therapy Studies, sponsored by the American Association of Physicists in Medicine, and supported by the National Cancer Institute reviews the correctness of dose measurement and calculation for patients entered into interinstitutional clinical trials. This program operates on a national scale. The other program, sponsored initially by the American College of Radiology with support by the National Cancer Institute and then the Regional Medical Program, has as a primary goal the improvement in the practice of medical physics in Texas particularly in relation to radiation therapy. My purpose here is to try to draw conclusions from these experiences which may have implications for the operation of a cancer center. I will not review in detail the technical findings of these programs since they have been or will be published elsewhere [1]. The work has been done by a number of people whose names appear in the acknowledgment.

The Radiological Physics Center – Operation

The Radiological Physics Center has reviewed the dosimetry at 85 institutions participating in 11 interinstitutional trial groups. The principal method of review is by visit to the institution by a physicist where measurements, calculations and techniques are reviewed. In one study a consulting radiotherapist and physicist visit the institution together. From the visit a judgment as to the correctness of the dosimetry system relating to the clinical trials is made. In most of the studies the dosimetry records of individual patients are reviewed to determine whether the prescribed radiation tumor dose has been fulfilled to within $\pm$ 5%, the criterion of acceptability. Where errors in the dosimetry system or discrepancies in the fulfillment of tumor dose exceed the criteria, the Radiological Physics Center works with institutions to clear misunderstandings or to rectify the errors.

Texas Regional Medical Physicists – Operation

The Texas Regional Medical Physicists is an organization of the 43 medical physicists in Texas (and a few from surrounding states) whose purpose is to improve the quality of medical physics which individual physicists offer to the medical profession. Current activities are listed in table I. During the last 2 years 1,600 individual patient dose distributions have been made and 400 of the other activities have occurred. In the last year dosimetry reviews have been made for 24 machines at 18 institutions. It is to be emphasized that the visits are at the request of and with the institution physicist; this activity should be considered an educational experience rather than a continuing service commitment.

Table I. Activities of the Texas regional medical physicists and the Regional Calibration Laboratory

---

1. Instrument calibration (Regional Calibration Laboratory)
2. Dosimetry reviews with individual physicists at their institution
3. System of mailed thermoluminescent dosimeters
4. System of mailed films for verifying uniformity of radiation beams and their coincidence with the light localizer pattern
5. Telecopier network to receive data and return dose distribution calculations for individual patients
6. Rental of expensive but infrequently used equipment such as anatomic phantoms
7. Monthly list of citations of pertinent new literature
8. Semi-annual workshops
9. Maintain and distribute lists of members who are available for physics consultation (as individuals)

At the onset, it was agreed that individual physicists would be responsible for the correctness of their own work. A possible exception was item 9 in table I in which inclusion of a physicist on a list of consultants might imply endorsement by the association for the individual. In 6 categories in which physicists are listed as available for consultation, only in therapy machine calibration is there substantial risk of injury to patients. In order to have some protection to the association it was agreed by the membership that those physicists listed as consultants for the calibration of therapy machines were obligated to use mailed thermoluminescent dosimeters for verification of calibrations (item 3, table I).

Another area of concern was the possibility that the activities of the central office might intrude into the relationship between the individual physicist and the radiotherapist or radiologist, perhaps thus diminishing the effectiveness of that team. This intrusion has not happened. At the present time 94% of the transactions of the central office are with physicists and not directly with physicians.

To date, there has been a fair measure of success in the standardization in the measurement of radiation dose and a consistency of dose calculation methods. In addition, the telecopier network can communicate graphical material between any station. There has been one radiotherapist in private practice who communicates with about 5 radiologists on clinical matters. The larger radiotherapy installations have used the communications system in only a minor way thus far. However, the system is available for clinical communication between any two stations with some assurance that the radiological physics at the two ends is consistent.

The program no longer has federal support and is, or is just about, self-supporting.

Findings

The technical findings from the two programs were almost the same. About 80% of the machines were delivering doses to within $\pm 5\%$ of that prescribed. Those that did not ranged from $+21$ to -47%. All but a few of the problems have been corrected as of this time. The nature, frequency and magnitude of the problems (but not the identity of the institutions) have been communicated to the radiological community at large [1]. The clinical importance of differences in dose of 5–10% has been demonstrated in some types of radiotherapy [3], and [2] and will not be elaborated upon here.

Conclusions

Some of the generalized conclusions which may be useful in the cancer center concept are:

1. In radiological physics and probably in radiation therapy there is need for an interinstitutional quality control mechanism. In some of the institutions which failed to meet the $\pm 5\%$ criterion in the fulfillment of tumor dose, the quality of physics staff was excellent.

2. Workshops, protocols, scientific meetings are helpful but not sufficient to assure sound techniques. Physicists making measurements and calculations together transmit information to each other. It is probable that radiotherapists must see patients together to transmit techniques effectively.

3. Physicists and radiotherapists are receptive to suggestions. In the early clinical trials care was taken to avoid offending radiotherapists by suggesting techniques; but experience has revealed that participating therapists were eager for suggestions.

4. Radiotherapists and physicists were objective and professional in understanding and rectifying errors at their institution. The early concerns about not injuring professional feelings were largely unnecessary.

5. Interinstitutional clinical trials can have an important educational function in addition to their stated research objectives.

6. Interinstitutional trials produce a demand for clarity and detail in the statement of methods which may result in improved standards of performance.

7. Cooperative activities require patience. Progress in improved standards in Texas which were expected in 1 year required about 4 years. Clinical collaboration which is very much more complex than collaboration in physics will likely require much time and labor.

Observations

There have been prolonged and unresolved arguments in committee meetings on the question: 'Is it better for the patient if advanced centers (a) ignore, or (b) try to collaborate with institutions practicing radiation therapy in which the equipment and/or skill of the physicians is limited?' I do not know the answer but have found myself arguing on the side of (b). I suggest the following principle for considering the above question:

Treat every patient above some acceptable
standard of quality for his type and stage
of disease near his home if that is possible;
if that is not possible, refer the patient
to an institution able to offer adequate
treatment.

This is not a new principle, but one which is roughly operative in medicine. Radiotherapy and radiological physics do not have acceptable standards defined at this time. However, a start in this direction has been made in the protocols of interinstitutional clinical trials. There is probably little objection to the principle above; however, there may be questions as to whether it can be implemented. It seems to me there should be at least three features in the implementation: (1) agreement concerning which patients will be treated where; (2) a flow of information, consultation and instruction, and (3) movement of patients where appropriate to fulfill the agreement in (1).

There is residual opinion that cooperative programs will not work. Accordingly, there will be a willingness to point to early failures or rebuffs to support that view. I think that physicians undertaking cooperative activities should realize that a very long time may be required – perhaps a decade – to see tangible results and that a system is likely to be fragile and require continuing attention. The magnitude of the effort may require professional sacrifice in less research accomplished, fewer papers published and less recognition on a national scale. Yet there is the possibility, if one perseveres, that through cooperative efforts such as cancer centers the average quality of patient treatment will improve and that academic institutions will have a sufficient number of appropriate cases within the system for the training of young physicians.

Acknowledgment

Grateful acknowledgment is made to MARILYN STOVALL, ALFRED SMITH, WALTER GRANT, ROBERT GOLDEN, JACKSON CUNDIFF and WILLIAM STOREY for performing the bulk of the work referred to in the text.

This work was supported in part by grant CA 10953 from the National Cancer Institute and grant RM 00007 from the Regional Medical Program.

References

1 GOLDEN, R.; CUNDIFF J. H.; GRANT, W. H. and SHALEK, R. J.: A review of the activities of the AAPM Radiological Physics Center in interinstitutional trials involving radiation therapy. Cancer, Philad. *29:* 1468–1472 (1972).
2 HERRING, D. F.: The degree of precision required in the radiation dose delivered in cancer radiotherapy. Report No. EMI-216 (Enviro-Med Inc., La Jolla 1970).
3 SHUKOVSKY, L. J.: Dose, time, volume relationships in squamous cell carcinoma of the supraglottic larynx. Am. f. Roentgenol., Radium Therapy and Nucl. Med. *108:* 27 (1970).

Author's address: Dr. ROBERT J. SHALEK, The University of Texas at Houston, M. D. Anderson Hospital and Tumor Institute, Department of Physics, 6723 Bertner Avenue, *Houston, TX 77025* (USA)

Front. Radiation Ther. Onc., vol. 8, pp. 126–131
(Karger, Basel and University Park Press, Baltimore 1973)

Medical Oncology Training in the Cancer Center[1]

D. W. GOLDE and M. J. CLINE

Cancer Research Institute, University of California, San Francisco, Calif.

Introduction

Medical oncology, a relatively new discipline within the speciality of internal medicine, is currently in the process of defining its educational responsibilities and goals. The title 'medical oncologist' is preferable to 'chemotherapist' in that the latter term emphasizes only a limited aspect of the medical management of neoplastic disease. The medical oncologist is an internist who is specially trained to provide overall care for the cancer patient. This individual must be highly skilled in all phases of internal medicine and have extensive knowledge of tumor biology and the clinical pharmacology of anti neoplastic agents. He should be a competent hematologist and have a broad understanding of cancer surgery and radiation therapy. The medical oncologist needs particular ability to manage infectious disease, perform clinical procedures, and deal with the psychological needs of his patients and their families. He also must have the emotional maturity to relate daily with very sick patients and the organizational capacity to coordinate the multidisciplinary approach to cancer patient care. How is such an individual trained and what are the medical oncologist's responsibilities to provide training for students and personnel in related specialties?

1   Supported by USPMS Grant CA 11067.

Organization

Clearly, education and training in medical oncology can be effective only in a center which provides outstanding clinical care. The cancer unit must not only be complete in terms of facilities and personnel, but must also have the commitment to excellence in patient care which creates the necessary environment for learning. An absolute prerequisite for proper patient management is a close and informed working relationship between the medical oncologist, radiation therapist and cancer surgeon. Coordination and cooperation between these disciplines cannot rest on compatibility among individuals, but must be formalized in terms of unit structure, scheduling and grant support. Clinical and basic research within the unit provides depth to the training program and broadens the clinical experience.

In addition to the requirements for cancer patient care, the training unit needs special educational capability. At the Cancer Research Institute, for example, we have a full-time teacher-clinician who functions to coordinate and direct the educational activities of the unit. This individual is an outstanding clinical oncologist and teacher who holds faculty appointments in the Cancer Research Institute and Department of Medicine and has no significant research or administrative responsibilities. This position formalizes the commitment to education and provides focus and direction for the training program.

At the Cancer Research Institute we also maintain a complete hematology laboratory to provide rapid hematologic data for the clinic and to permit trainees and students to involve themselves directly and regularly in the laboratory hematology aspects of patient care. A qualified clinical pathologist supervises the laboratory and provides daily informal consultation as well as a structured program in bone marrow morphology. The staff also includes an anatomic pathologist who regularly reviews biopsy material with the clinical personnel. The educational responsibilities of the staff members are clearly delineated. Attending oncologists supervise the ward, clinic and consultation services on a rotating basis. Research seminars and chemotherapy protocol reviews are held regularly and there is an active and well-attended monthly journal club. A weekly teaching exercise is conducted at which the entire staff and local practicing oncologists review a case representing an important problem in clinical oncology. Lectures by guest speakers are given approximately every 2 weeks. Particular attention is paid to the teaching function of the weekly tumor board, and the active participation of students and trainees is encouraged.

Training of the Medical Oncologist

The ideal candidate for a medical oncology training program is an accomplished internist seeking sub-specialty experience in the management of neoplastic disease. Usually such an individual will have at least 2 years of training in internal medicine and may have had previous hematology and oncology experience. Clearly the educational program must be flexible enough to meet individual needs yet structured sufficiently to provide adequate exposure to the disciplines related to cancer patient management. To this end we allow the trainee to tailor the program to his career goals and to complement his previous training. Thus, for example, an individual with extensive previous hematology experience would waive the hematology rotation and perhaps select additional exposure to oncology research or radiation therapy. Similarly, an individual who is not research-oriented may select rotations in such clinically related areas as infectious disease or even psychiatry.

Generally, we believe a 2-year training period is required to properly prepare the specialist in medical oncology. The foundation of the program rests with the ward and clinic experience, and trainees usually spend a minimum of 6 months on the in-patient service. (The basic daily schedule for trainees on the ward service is shown in table I.) In addition, rotations are provided in adult and pediatric hematology, consultation service and radiation therapy. We consider a 2-month active and participatory rotation in radiation therapy to be a necessary part of the medical oncologist's training. Also, a number of electives in cancer surgery and various research areas are offered.

Training in Medical Oncology for the Radiation Therapist

Residents in radiation therapy spend at least 2 months on the clinical cancer ward where they follow a schedule identical to that of the medical oncology trainee. The radiation therapy resident benefits most importantly from the experience of providing primary medical care for the cancer patient. He also learns the fundamentals of cancer chemotherapy. Cooperation and understanding between the radiation therapist and medical oncologist is established at the trainee level.

This year we have also undertaken to provide training for the radiation therapy intern. His needs are unique in that he has had no clinical experience

Table I. Daily schedule for trainees on the Ward Service Cancer Research Institute, University of California, San Francisco

08.00 h						
	Ward rounds	Ward rounds	Ward rounds	Ward rounds	Ward rounds	Ward rounds
09.30 h						
			CRI conference		Attending rounds	
		X-ray conference		X-ray conference		
10.30 h						
	Attending rounds	Attending rounds	Medical grand rounds	Attending rounds	Tumor board	
12.00 h						
	Noon medical conference	Hematology-oncology conference	Protocol review and chemo-therapy seminar	Noon medical conference	Research seminar	
13.00 h						
		CRI Clinic		CRI Clinic	Pathology and bone marrow conference	
16.00 h						
	Radio-therapy conference	Radio-therapy conference	Radio-therapy conference	Radio-therapy conference	Radio-therapy conference	

as a graduate physician. Within the present system the radiation therapy interns spend 6 months on the clinical cancer service and 3 months on gynecology and otolaryngology. This program is designed to provide a fundamental experience in the medical care of patients with neoplastic disease and exposure to the surgical sub-specialty areas with which the radiation therapist is particularly concerned.

Student Training

Medical students at the University of California, San Francisco, who elect the oncology pathway course are offered instruction in all disciplines related to the care of cancer patients. The students are divided into groups which rotate through the in-patient service, out-patient clinics, radiation therapy and cancer surgery. A 1-week elective period is provided to allow the student to pursue a particular area of interest. The students participate in the regular activities of the cancer unit; however, special faculty supervision is provided to insure proper instruction at the student level. Thus, patient reviews are conducted with the students in small groups as a function separate from the ward or clinic routine in order to facilitate the presentation of basic clinical oncology principles in a manner tailored to the needs of 3rd- and 4th-year medical students. The educational inadequacy of simply allowing students to participate on a good clinical service are well-known and it is prudent to periodically review the aspects of the program which are directed primarily toward education at the medical student level.

The students meet as a full group once daily for teaching seminars. The seminars are conducted by a faculty member and a student discussant who is responsible for a specific aspect of the subject to be covered. This format encourages general student participation and gives the student discussant the opportunity to explore a specific area of oncology in depth. The seminars

Table II. Representative student seminar topics

Viral carcinogenesis; implications for man
Cell cycle, cell replication and tumor growth
Hormones and carcinoma of the breast
Pharmacology of cancer chemotherapeutic agents
Mechanisms of radiation action
Hemopoietic cell replication and hematologic malignancies
The radiosensitive tumors; clinical management
Lymphocyte effector substances and tumor cell destruction by immunocytes
Primary management – breast
Tumor pathology
Impaired host; microbial killing mechanisms and clinical syndromes
Melanoma: head and neck tumors
Management of medical emergencies in oncology
Hodgkin's disease and lymphosarcoma; pathology, spread and staging
Lymphoma treatment
Psychological and social problems in oncology

are informal and are normally held during the lunch hour. A list of representative seminar subjects is shown in table II.

Evaluation

To be effective, evaluation should be an integral part of the educational process and must occur concomitantly with the training function. At the Cancer Research Institute, meetings are held every 2 weeks with the trainees to evalute the program. In addition to general topics related to the overall training structure, specific problems are openly discussed and acted upon. Decisions and changes in the training program are made as a direct consequence of this feedback. The instructors are also evaluated and responsibilities are assigned in a manner consistent with past performance.

Summary

The medical oncologist is an internist who is expert in the management of neoplastic disease. The cancer unit must be equipped and staffed to provide outstanding care for the cancer patient as a basic requirement for a training program in clinical oncology. Special organization, however, is necessary to provide effective education, and it is desirable to have a full-time teacher-clinician to direct and coordinate the training function. The program must be structured to meet specific needs for training the medical oncologist, radiation therapist and medical student, yet provide sufficient flexibility to be responsive to individual needs. Evaluation should be part of the educational process, occur concomitantly with the training function, and be translated rapidly into improved education.

Authors' address: Dr. DAVID W. GOLDE and Dr. MARTIN J. CLINE, Cancer Research Institute, University of California Medical Center, *San Francisco, CA 94122* (USA)

Front. Radiation Ther. Onc., vol. 8, pp. 132–134
(Karger, Basel and University Park Press, Baltimore 1973)

Training in the Cancer Center

Radiation Therapy

J. P. GREEN

West Coast Cancer Foundation, and St. Francis Memorial Hospital,
San Francisco, Calif.

Education must be considered a basic function of the cancer center radiation therapy department. The training of radiation therapy residents is still the core of the educational program of such a department, but with the continued development of this specialty, as well as the multidisciplinary approach to cancer, knowledge of radiation therapy becomes mandatory for a multitude of others. The purpose of this paper is to point out where this exposure is required, and to discuss possible educational approaches.

I. Radiation Therapy Personnel

A. Graduate and Undergraduate Levels
1. Residents and interns. To discuss the format of residency training programs is not the intent of this meeting, but the establishment of the radiation therapy internship is worth mentioning. Interns must be recruited directly from medical school and obtained through the matching program, in competition with all other existing internships. The internship requires a close working relationship with the other departments of the center, as 6 months of electives are included in the 1-year curriculum. The center and department must, of course, be able to offer an American Medical Association accredited program.

2. Externs. A clinical oncology clerkship program was initiated by our group in 1966. To date, a total of 30 students has participated. Third- and fourth-year medical students from schools across the country have been selected annually to participate in an 8-week program.

The aim of the program is to orient the students to clinical oncology. Emphasis is placed on a proper understanding of the basic problems rather than on the technical aspects of surgery or radiation therapy.

Any student spending 8 weeks in the clerkship will be more sophisticated and knowledgeable in the field of oncology, making it a worthwhile experience regardless of what specialty he ultimately selects. Because of the national shortage of oncologic physicians, the value of the program is reflected in the number of students who decide on a career in oncology. Six of our past students are presently in our residency training program. In all, 11 of the 30 have chosen the field of oncology for their future work.

3. Technicians. Radiation therapy technology training is essential to provide adequate numbers of qualified personnel in this area. Training should be on a high intellectual level, including courses in physics and biology. It has been our experience that much of the training can be given simultaneously to junior-level resident physicians and student technologists, thereby avoiding duplication of efforts.

II. Radiation Therapy Personnel, Postgraduate

A. Radiation Therapists
The center should be available to those practitioners desirous of returning to an academic environment for refreshment of techniques and philosophy. The physician actually participating in a working situation is provided with a different perspective and experience than that received from attendance at national meetings.

B. General Radiologists
Although fully trained therapists will eventually assume the full responsibility for radiation therapy in this country, general radiologists are still very much involved in such practises. Their continued education, both at the center and in their home communities should be ardently pursued.

C. Technicians
Therapy technicians in practice require periodic refreshment to maintain a level of expertise and to keep up with newer techniques. This again should be provided by the center.

III. Nonradiation Therapy Personnel

A. Medical Students

Medical students must have greater exposure to oncology, including radiotherapy, which heretofore in most centers was negligible. Lecture-seminar time, electives and a tour of the department for all students, regardless of ultimate career goals, must be made available.

B. Dental Students

These students in our recent experience have proven enthusiastic recipients of training in oncology and radiation therapy. The benefits to the community from having cancer-knowledgeable dentists are obvious. Teaching includes third- and fourth-year lecture series (4–6 h) and attendance at the head and neck conference, and weekly patient rounds (4 h).

C. Medical Oncology Residents

A full understanding of radiation therapy is necessary for medical oncologists. An uninterrupted block of time in the radiation therapy department is strongly recommended – 3 months being a reasonable period of time. In addition, attendance at ongoing rounds and conferences should be encouraged.

D. Surgical and Surgical Subspecialty Residents

This is a less well defined area as there are few surgeons being trained exclusively in oncology. However, any surgeon expecting to devote a portion of his practise to oncology should have more than casual exposure to radiation therapy. One rewarding experience has been with a gynecologic residency in the Bay Area, where third-year residents spend one full month in the radiation therapy department – participating in all departmental teaching activities, but with the emphasis on gynecologic cancer.

E. General Medical Profession

So-called 'grass-roots' education of the general medical profession is essential to the overall concept of upgrading cancer management in any community. The departmental staff should be available to the peripheral community hospitals and medical staffs for tumor boards, lectures, conferences, etc.

Author's address: Dr. JEROLD P. GREEN, West Coast Cancer Foundation, Department of Radiation Therapy, St. Francis Memorial Hospital, 900 Hyde Street, *San Francisco, CA 94109* (USA)

Front. Radiation Ther. Onc., vol. 8, pp. 135–138
(Karger, Basel and University Park Press, Baltimore 1973)

Training in the Cancer Center – Integration III

Surgery

R. V. De Vito

University of Washington, Seattle, Wash.

Introduction

Possibly the most important recent advance in cancer management is represented by the increased communication between those specialties involved in the treatment of malignant tumors. It is refreshing that fewer meetings are restricted to the surgery of cancer, or radiation therapy of cancer or chemotherapy of cancer, while more are devoted to the *management* of cancer. With such communication, capable and conscientious physicians have developed a sometimes surprised awareness of what various modalities have to offer, an appreciation that all specialities are interdependent and a sense of mutual respect. Old jealousies and prejudices are being discarded in favor of a comfortable system of open cooperation.

In the 19th century, heroic surgical forays were waged against cancer, with none of the many advantages relied upon for the simplest of operations today. It is not surprising that, for head and neck malignant tumors, radiation therapy became the modality of choice during the first half of this century. Indeed, surgeons such as MARTIN, MacCOMB and CADE became radiation therapists. During World War II, however, surgical daring combined with improved anesthetic techniques, better fluid therapy including blood transfusions, and the advent of antibiotics to initiate an era of surgical preeminence in the management of malignant tumors of the skin and of the head and neck. It is unfortunate that surgeons of the past 25-30 years have been slow in realizing that similarly significant advances were being made in radiation therapy, chemotherapy and immunotherapy. Nonetheless, such realization is now becoming more commonplace and will hopefully become routine.

Concepts Involved

The surgeon's role in an integrated cancer center, exept for his unique technical capabilities, is no different to that of all physicians in the center. Each should be reasonably talented and aggressive in his or her specific field. A conscientious physician – no matter how open-minded – will not 'give up' his patient unless assured that excellent management is available, and the team will fail if old habits of protective possessiveness are not abandoned. Respect for one's capabilities develops only when performance justifies respect. Secondly, each individual must be capable of learning from another; each must be secure enough that a team concept is not threatening, honest and humble enough to admit shortcomings, and scientific enough to accept factual data. Thirdly, the team members must be capable, individually and collectively, in their rôle as teachers. This requires not only didactic ability but an emotional and philosophical commitment; the surgeon for example, will be required to teach 'his techniques' to competing specialties, to control surgical trainees in their enthusiasm for operation, and to support other specialties in teaching sessions. Fourthly, one must be capable of working within a structured environment of collaboration. The various clinical 'workshops' must be physically and philosophically accessible to all, and the physical plant and mechanics of staffing should be such that it is more convenient, efficient, and productive for the team to work *together*. This collaboration must include evaluation and treatment of patients, critical episodic analysis of treatment plans and treatment results, clinical and laboratory research, and all aspects of the teaching program.

Mechanisms at the University of Washington

The mechanisms established for training in cancer at the University of Washington in Seattle have evolved over a number of years, Firstly, all formal oncology teaching sessions for students in the School of Medicine are done on a conjoint basis. House staff conferences and continuing medical education courses are similarly collaborative. Secondly, a number of tumor clinics has been established. The Head and Neck Clinic, for example, is held weekly. In regular attendance at this clinic are staff men and residents in radiation therapy, plastic and general surgery, otolaryngology, oral surgery and medical oncology. Patients from all four teaching hospitals in the University of Washington system and from outside referrals are evaluated and followed in this one clinic. Medical and dental students attend regularly. Similar integrated clinics, with appropriate staffing, include a lymphoma clinic, a gynecologic clinic, a breast cancer clinic and the urology cancer conference. Thirdly, the University Clinical Cancer Group has been established. This was done partly to 'bring into the fold' the few remaining isolationists on the faculty (true believers always become missionaries), but primarily to improve the caliber of patient care and the level of service to patients and physicians of the regional community. All medical school and dental school departments and all individual physicians and dentists involved in cancer patient care – diagnosis, acute management, chronic care, rehabilitation, *et cetera* – were, and are, invited to participate.

The objectives of this group are best summarized by the announcement distributed at its inception:

'This is to announce the available services of the *University Clinical Cancer Group*, a multidisciplinary university hospital group of clinicians with primary commitment to the care of cancer patients. Each of the departments involved in caring for such patients has been invited to participate in activities of the group; approximately 15 clinicians have been active in organization of the group and formulating policies.

The *University Clinical Cancer Group* has one guiding principle – provision of the best possible patient care. Other objectives are as follows:

1. To offer a specific identifiable clinical unit for consultations and referrals from outside physicians.

2. To attract a larger number of cancer patients to this institution, facilitating successful clinical research. This is presently hampered in part by inadequate numbers of patients.

3. To develop more effective training programs for clinicians managing cancer programs.

4. To contribute to community education in the northwest.

The group offers a service not currently available in this region. Physicians who care for cancer patients as inpatients or outpatients at the university hospital will have the option of requesting a 'cancer consultation'. Such a request will be received by the administrative assistant, who will arrange for appropriate clinicians representing various specialties to see the patient together. By this means the patient will receive a more comprehensive consultation without the days of waiting for consultations as in the past. This will be a saving of time and money for the patient. The charge to the patient will be lower than individual consultations because a flat fee for the group will be arranged.

Existing prerogatives of the university physicians will remain the same. The physician caring for a patient will remain in charge. He does not need to request the services of the group, nor does he need to accept its recommendations or to relinquish care of the patient. In general, consultations by this group will be carried out the same day in which requests are received.'

The administrative assistant plays a crucial rôle; a daily cancer activity data sheet is distributed which summarizes all pathology examinations of cancer tissue, all inpatient admissions with a cancer diagnosis, and all new pertinent outpatient clinic appointments. All group consults are summarized on a monthly basis, episodic statistical reviews for specific lesions or services are tabulated, and monthly meetings of the entire group are held to evaluate progress.

Lectures and seminars are coordinated so that a conjoint presentation by multiple disciplines is made whenever possible. The Department of Continuing Medical Education uses the central office as a clearing house for speaker requests, and in arranging postgraduate courses sponsored by the department or by the Regional Medical Program. Again, whenever feasible, an interdependent, cooperative, multidisciplinary approach to cancer is stressed in these presentations.

Intelligent management of cancer requires an integrated approach to diagnosis, treatment and rehabilitation. It is an over-riding obligation of those involved in teaching programs to impart this concept to trainees. The surgeon learns by doing, and teaches by showing; the surgeon who wishes to teach in a cancer center must, therefore, participate actively and enthusiastically in a truly cooperative program.

Author's address: Dr. R. V. De Vito, University of Washington, 1959 Pacific Avenue, *Seattle, WA 98105* (USA)

Front. Radiation Ther. Onc., vol. 8, pp. 139–144
(Karger, Basel and University Park Press, Baltimore 1973)

The Relationship of Basic Research
to a Cancer Center

R. O. Lowy

West Coast Cancer Foundation, and Department of Radiation Therapy,
St. Vincent's Hospital, Portland, Oregon

Closely coordinated clinical and research units are the foundation of a true cancer center. In such an atmosphere, both may achieve their primary objective for the production of maximum results for the greatest benefit to the cancer patient. In the ideal situation, a cancer center is one which has a strong clinical unit and an equally strong research unit, conjoined with either a medical school or medical center. In reality, a center usually begins with either a strong clinical or research facility which would initially predetermine the goals of research, the lines of communication and the physical plant. The following will be a presentation of the research program for a cancer center whose stress is in the clinical therapeutic management of the cancer patient (fig. 1).

In the past, basic research has been conducted relatively free from great financial restrictions or social pressures. Currently, our resources necessary for scientific investigation appear to be limited and it becomes our responsibility to find more efficient means of research, as well as the means for applying the vast accumulated stores of information. Yet, in spite of the great concerted effort of researchers attempting to elucidate the nature, prevention and cure of malignant disease, there is still fundamental information lacking which will be required in order to effectively control cancer. It is in this quest that a multidisciplinary approach to the basic oncobiologic nature of cancer is directed. Therefore, within the research unit of a cancer center, there should be individuals dedicated not only to the discovery of new basic information but to its application and dissemination. This is not to deny the scientist the freedom to do basic research, but to invest in him a social conscience in return for the privileges of financial support and ego recognition given to him by our society.

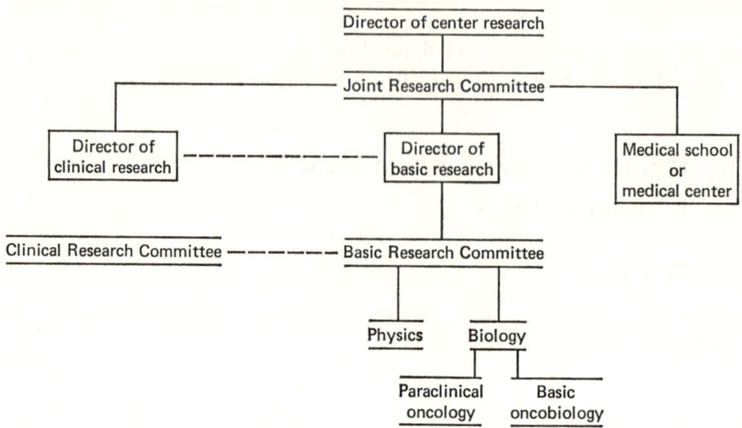

Fig. 1. Administrative Organization

Before this past decade, cancer therapies have developed along empirical lines, by trial and error, for the convenience of the therapist, and have been limited by the therapeutic modalities available. More sophisticated and rational cancer treatment now appears to be possible if the results of research can be transformed from the controlled laboratory environment to the human situation. Unfortunately, in the past when the clinical observation was taken to the laboratory, lines of investigation developed that required the creation of a highly artificial tumor model. Attempts to learn more about the tumor model have created divergent lines of investigation until the clinical situation was lost in the fervor and excitement of new discoveries of the artificial model system. Attempts of the brave few to extrapolate this data back to the clinical problem have brought skepticism from both the clinician and the laboratory scientist.

Within the development of a cancer center, the key individual is the director of all cancer research, both clinical and fundamental. This individual should be a physician of extraordinary qualities, capable of envisioning the entire scope of cancer research and having the ability to mobilize and direct the resources of the center along well developed lines of productive investigation. In order to coordinate the interests of the center, he will be chairman of the joint research committee. Comembers will be representatives from the 3 major center units, individuals from other local scientific institutions and qualified private citizens representing the community at large. It will be this committee's major responsibility to develop the guidelines for research and coordinate the growth and development of the research program for the center.

In the initial development of a research program in a clinically oriented cancer center, the emphasis on research activity will reflect the needs and interests of the clinical group. With the inception of each joint research project, the basic science component will itself be developed to furnish the necessary fundamental research and productive potential. In this manner, the basic oncobiologic science division will enlarge to meet the research needs of the center.

Meaningful and efficient investigation will be achieved if the research program of the center accepts the concept of limited numbers of areas of investigation, stressing interdisciplinary, in-depth research. It is impossible to cover all areas of cancer research. With an active clinical unit and a well rounded medical center, it will become evident that there are certain areas of research and expertise which will result by interaction of the 3 units. No area of research should be undertaken merely because it is in vogue unless one has specially trained individuals and facilities to make a significant contribution.

For each major research project, both clinician and scientist would be jointly responsible for presenting the proposed project and organizing those research disciplines required for the many aspects of investigation. These individuals would either actively participate in the joint research activities or act as coadvisors.

The basic research unit would consist of the basic oncobiologic sciences and applied research of radiobiology, chemobiology, immunology and experimental cancer surgery, and would be ideally suited to a centralized physical plant. This would facilitate interdepartmental communication and reduce duplications of both equipment and effort. The basic science core facilities should be in proximity to the area of experimental clinical research of the cancer center. For radiation therapy, this may consist of new particle accelerators; and for chemotherapy and immunotherapy, facilities to carry out new means of therapeutics with patient care support and chemical and immunologic laboratories.

Research policies and goals would be set forth by the basic research committee composed of the director of research and representatives from divisions of physics research, paraclinical experimental research and basic oncobiologic research. This committee would meet on a regular basis with the clinical research committee. This joint review committtee would be responsible for approving new research applications which would contain

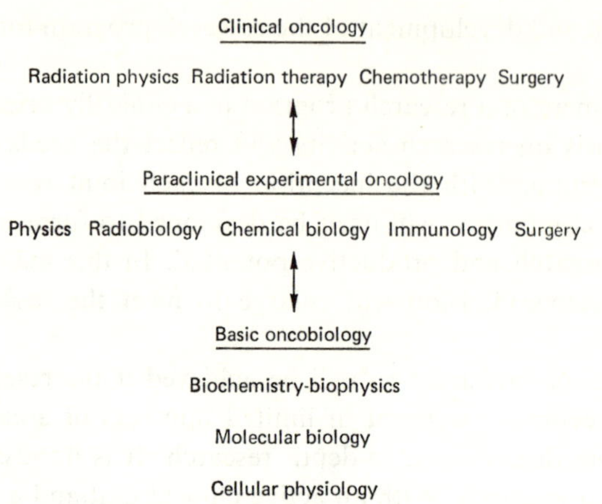

Fig. 2. Research Organization.

complete detailed information concerning the project goals, materials and methods, personnel requirements for investigation, financial expenditures and the length of the projects. Projects underway will be expected to report research progress. In addition, the joint research-clinical commitee will have responsibility for reviewing grant applications for individual investigators, and for the research unit.

Within the physics division, research would be conducted in both the applied and fundamental level, closely coordinated with biologic and clinical research projects. Biologic research involving irradiation would require cooperative participation with the physics division. The individual appointed to head the physics research would be one who was knowledgeable in both the clinically applied and basically oriented aspects of research. He must be able to appreciate the fundamental problems in clinical radiation therapy and be available for treatment planning consultation.

The biologic research division would contain two separate organizational levels: the paraclinical experimental and the basic oncobiologic (fig. 2). Biologic research would cover a much wider range than those interacting with the physics section, involving all of the clinical oncologic specialities. Each of these organization levels would initially be developed by the needs of the research center to conduct joint investigational projects. The individual scientists needed at each level would be required to have different degrees of involvement in the clinically oriented projects. This would be dependent upon their own qualifications and interests, as well as the needs of the projects. Those scientists with clinical exposure and orientation naturally would be the senior investigators of joint projects and would need scientists under them who could devote themselves full-time to basic research.

Communications within the physics and biology divisions would occur during frequent (i.e., weekly) administrative and scientific meetings. Their purpose would be to plan research activities for each week. Communication between the research divisions and the clinical unit would be effected through monthly joint seminars and research meetings. Clinical sessions appraising results of specific modalities of treatment and morbidity of therapy would be attended by both clinician and basic scientist. It would be through these meetings that new clinical problems could be evaluated directly with the applied biologic investigator and possible avenues of basic research discussed. In addition, basic science seminars would be arranged which would present data in areas of basic investigation with potential for application to actual clinical oncology.

Finally, the cancer center should plan for the publication of a scientific journal to include papers on clinical investigation, basic oncologic research and those most important projects including cooperative interdisciplinary investigation.

Though the stress of the center is on cooperative research, this is not to deny the scientist the opportunity for independent individual investigations. Adequate time, facilities and financial support should be made available for relevant areas of oncologic investigation. Scientists should consider time and efforts equally divided between independent research, joint research and teaching commitments.

The teaching commitment should include a didactic lecture series and laboratory exercises in both biologic and physical sciences, and should be tailored to the trainees' level of education and experience as well as their professional needs. Postgraduate programs leading to advanced degrees should be developed in the various basic oncologic subspecialities and offered to those individuals with B.S. and M.D. qualifications. In addition to the lecture and laboratory series, some research experiences should be incorporated into the training program. Postgraduate residency training in radiation therapy, chemotherapy or surgery should include 6–12 months of full-time laboratory research. Ideally, these projects should be stimulated by the individuals' personal clinical experience, and they should be guided to formulate and develop the specific format and details of research. They should be given specific instruction in the theories of experimental design, laboratory animal techniques, tumor models and statistical analysis. These projects should be of such quality as to merit formal presentations and preparations of a scientific manuscript for publication.

Summary

The integration of a multidisciplined, basic research unit is a major goal in the building of a successful cancer center. Basic research is multidisciplined in the organization of applied and basic oncobiology, and in its fundamental research into the biologic nature of cancer and application and utilization of this knowledge for the patient. Major research projects should be limited in number and wide in the scope and the depth of research; they should be generated through the needs of the clinical, therapeutic management of the patient. The basic science teaching program will include the training of basic scientists, oncologists and paramedical personnel through well organized lecture series, laboratory exercises and practical research experience.

Author's address: Dr. R. O. Lowy, Department of Radiation Therapy, St. Vincent's Hospital, *Portland, Oreg.* (USA)

Front. Radiation Ther. Onc., vol. 8, pp. 145–174
(Karger, Basel and University Park Press, Baltimore 1973)

Multidiscipline Clinical Trials in Cancer Centers[1]

P. RUBIN

Division of Therapeutic Radiology, Strong Memorial Hospital,
University of Rochester, Rochester, N. Y.

I. Introduction

The mechanism for the integration of a radiation center into a cancer center is the clinical investigational program. The controlled trial is the generative mechanism for advances in clinical practice. There is a gradual realization by oncologists that the quality and quantity of a life afflicted by cancer can be improved. Formulating innovative approaches to cancer care does not provide a critical means to assess the new methods. One justification for centralization of radiation equipment is that it will concentrate personnel and patients and set the stage for investigative study. In the ideal circumstance, the clinical practice of therapeutic radiology or radiation oncology is enhanced by the developments in research.

The radiation center often is the beginning or major focus in cancer centers. The functional nature of its existence rests in a flow pattern of referral from all major medical and surgical specialties. It is multidisciplinary in its orientation toward cancer management. The translation of unidisciplinary trials of cancer surgery or cancer chemotherapy into combinations of methods can be accomplished best in radiation centers, for the quality of practice is high and specialization in radiotherapy groups develops and corresponds with major blocks of referred patients. Progress in cancer care will emerge from this multiple disciplined effort if identifiable obstacles can be overcome.

1   This study was supported by USPHS Grants CA-11051-05 and CA-12262-01.

II. *Obstacles to Multidisciplinary Clinical Trials*

The development of the radiation centers is essential to overcoming the following obstacles.

1. Development of many small operational units in therapeutic radiology outstrips available manpower. The proliferation of cobalt units in community hospitals has rapidly supplanted the orthovoltage unit. At one time there was a contraction of practice of therapeutic radiology to fewer hospitals with the abandonment of kilovoltage apparatus by many private practioners of general radiology. Presently, the number of supervoltage units, which includes both telecobalt equipment and accelerators, far exceeds the number of fully qualified therapeutic radiologists and ancillary personnel, such as physicists and dosimetrists. The improvement in treatment planning has created a demand for highly trained individuals to provide precise dosimetry. This requires computers, isodose curves, machine shops for special shields, devices, wedges, etc. This team of special personnel can best be realized in a radiation center and is essential to conducting accurate clinical trials.

2. There is a diffusion of patient experience by the desire of each community hospital to be independent and fully capable in all specialties. Larger numbers of certain types of patients are required to conduct clinical trials. Again, separate hospitals with individual therapy units morcellate a clinical experience. The creation of multi-unit radiation centers is desirable even if such units are geographically spaced. The clinical study can be a mechanism for achieving closer cooperation. Unless such cooperative studies are done, it will be impossible to accumulate an adequate series. The centralization of equipment, however, leads also to centralization of patients as well as trained personnel.

3. Attitudinal awareness of the importance of clinical trials is lacking. There is mixed feeling by many physicians as to the merits of clinical trials as a valid form of clinical investigation. There are ethical questions as to the utilization of one form of therapy as compared to another more conservative or radical approach. To overcome such questions, carefully designed studies are essential but it is important to develop a 'clinical research nucleus'. To expect a practitioner of radiation therapy to find time to fill in forms and follow detailed protocols is unrealistic. A senior member of the group of therapeutic radiologists should divide the responsibility among others on the staff and direct the program. A study secretary and a forms specialist are essential to data recording and checking. Perhaps the most difficult hurdle is the loss of the physician's decision-making in randomized trials where the choice of treatment is done remotely. Again, a collective of research personnel provides the proper attitude, and the environment of a radiation center is appropriate to this task.

4. Lack of precise data on results in cancer treatment. The diversification of treatment centers demands an integration of data and its retrieval. This problem is likely to be solved. There is a need for similar records to be kept, vital data stored in computers and retrieved for use in decision making. With the development of radiation centers an effort to coordinate is bound to occur. It can reinforce the present tendency to perform in individualistic ways by requiring a similar record system. Cooperation in a national network of radiation centers presupposes the development of such regional cancer centers.

5. The unidisciplinary decision-making process in cancer management can be a major hindrance. The most difficult block to clinical investigation is patient-ownership by the first physician to consult on a patient. This takes the form of the 'doctor-patient' relationship, a 'sacred cow' in the practice of medicine. A multidisciplinary approach is essential to cancer management. The clinical trial is the beginning of group decision-making. The acceptance of exploring a number of options in a coordinated fashion is the beginning of cooperative study, both at home and on the national level.

III. Clinical Trials by Theme

There are numerous clinical trials in cancer therapeutics and emerging radiation centers will not lack protocols. Analysis of clinical investigative themes can provide an insight into those areas of study given a high priority by present cooperative groups in existence. This can provide a basis for choice as to how such studies will be conducted. A brief outline of available themes to study is offered according to unidisciplinary and multidisciplinary efforts.

A. Unidisciplinary

1. Surgery. Comparison of techniques with simple *versus* radical approach or radical *versus* super-radical procedures often includes greater nodal dissections. Sites under study include breast cancer, lung cancer and cervix cancer.

2. Radiation therapy. There are a large number of studies evolving utilizing different tumor doses and treatment fractionation regimens. (a) Fractionation: split course is most popular theme under study in head and neck sites, bladder and cervix. (b) Oxygen breathing: hyperbaric and carbogen ($5\% \ CO_2$) are under study in lung, cervix, head and neck, brain. (c) Extended field: particularly for greater lymph node coverage in: Hodgkin's disease, leukemia, head and neck, bone, lymphosarcoma. (d) Quality of beam: this applies to higher energies, 25–40 MeV, electrons. (e) Special particles: high LET as neutrons, protons and Π-mesons. (f) Optimization of therapy: search for tumor dose and fractionation schedules which provide the most local tumor ablations and least complications.

3. Chemotherapy. (a) New agents are explored, namely in advanced, recurrent and metastatic disease. (b) Combinations of chemotherapy are very actively being explored in leukemia, Hodgkin's disease, lymphoma, lung, ovary, colon and soft tissue sarcoma.

4. Immunotherapy. This form of treatment is newest and is usually done within single institutions with highly targeted tumor sites. Both non-specific and specific stimuli to immune systems are under study.

B. Multidisciplinary

1. Surgery *versus* radiation therapy: competitive approach is under study in cervix cancer stage IA, uterine fundus and bladder cancer.

2. Surgery *versus* surgery and postoperative irradiation.

3. Surgery *versus* preoperative irradiation and surgery is being explored in breast cancer, lung cancer, some head and neck cancers, cervix, esophagus, rectum, kidney and bladder cancer.

4. Surgery and chemotherapy is being studied in pediatric solid tumors as Wilm's and neuroblastoma.

5. Radiation therapy and chemotherapy is very actively being studied in breast, lung, head and neck sites, cervix, ovary, esophagus, prostate, bone, brain, Hodgkin's disease, lymphomas, leukemia, Wilm's and neuroblastoma.

6. Surgery plus irradiation plus chemotherapy or hormonotherapy is another active theme being studied in breast cancer, lung, head and neck, cervix, ovary, bladder, prostate, testes, bone, soft tissue, brain, Wilm's and neuroblastoma.

7. Immunotherapy plus standard therapies is being explored in melanoma.

IV. Multidisciplinary Clinical Trials at Specific Sites

The emergence of the controlled clinical trial as the core investigational program in cancer can be attributed to the clinical cancer investigation review committee of National Institute of Health (NIH). At first, they encouraged cooperative trials within single specialities such as chemotherapists, surgeons and hematologists, and at single cancer sites such as lung, breast and Hodgkin's disease groups. As groups were formed for each disease, conflicts of interest developed amongst different disciplines. To avoid these conflicts, multiprotocol groups have been organized within the last 5 years. Most single categorical groups have become interdisciplinary oncology groups in their design committees.

The radiation therapy community was the last of the specialty groups to be organized and still faces problems in developing and moving protocol studies into operational phases. The role of the radiation center is invaluable in allowing a group of therapeutic radiologists to redirect part of their clinical effort to problem-solving. A brief description of protocols at each site can be obtained upon review of the recent protocol abstracts by FLAMANT [11] listed in the files of the Union Internationale Contre le Cancer (UICC) involving radiation therapy. Review of protocols [16] from some of the major cooperative groups such as the Radiation Therapy Oncology Group (RTOG), the Eastern Cooperative Oncology Group (ECOG), the Gynecologic Oncology Group (GOG), the Genito-Urinary Oncology Group (GUOG), and the Children's Cancer Study Group A has also been done in the preparation of this manuscript.

A. Breast Cancer

The localized forms of breast cancer stages I and II are being studied from a variety of viewpoints: the most appropriate surgical procedure, the value of preoperative and postoperative irradiation, and the addition of chemotherapeutic and hormonal manipulation at the time of surgery. Such drugs as cyclophosphamide and 5-FU have been utilized. The failures of surgery and radiation therapy can be entered into single and multiple drug protocols. Most advanced cases are first treated by hormonal measures and then entered into such protocols.

In progress is the major national program in breast cancer, directed by BERNARD FISHER [10] of the National Surgical Adjuvant Breast Project. The design of the study is to determine the proper surgical treatment for female breast cancer and the benefits of supplemental radiation therapy. The basis for determining the target group is the status of the axilla in localized cancer masses. The therapeutic options are total mastectomy *versus* radical mastectomy with and without postoperative irradiation (McWhirter's technique) to 5,000 rads in 5 weeks (fig. 1). There is a slower entry of cases than anticipated.

Future projections rest upon the current interest for managing localized cancer by a trial of lumpectomy followed by radiation therapy. The results obtained by MUSTAKILLIO [19], RIGBY-JONES [23] and PETERS [21] are en-

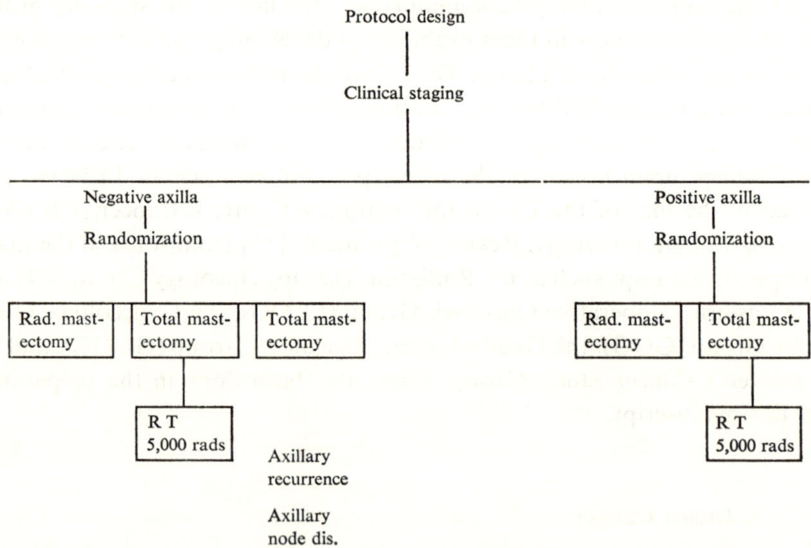

Fig. 1. Breast cancer, stages I and II. - National Surgical Adjuvant Breast Project. RT = radiation therapy. Total mastectomy = simple mastectomy (10).

couraging. Despite the interest of the therapeutic radiologist, it is unlikely that a national cooperative program will emerge until the more conservative total mastectomy is shown to be comparable to radical mastectomy. This conflict of interests can only be resolved by the disciplines that are in competition for the same block of patients working together and attempting to complete one study before starting another.

B. Lung Cancer

For intrapulmonary primary lung cancers with spread only to hilar nodes, the standard form of surgical treatment has been compared to the addition of pre- and postoperative irradiation, and single and multiple chemotherapy agents as cyclophosphamide, nitrogen mustard, vinblastine, 5-hydroxyurea, etc. For intrathoracic or extrathoracic extensions of lung cancer, single and multidrugs have been studied with small gain. The National Lung Task Force lead by OLEG SELAWRY [29] and the RTOG have been developing a series of protocols for all stages of lung cancer. The need for documentation of the most effective radiation therapy schedule in a variety

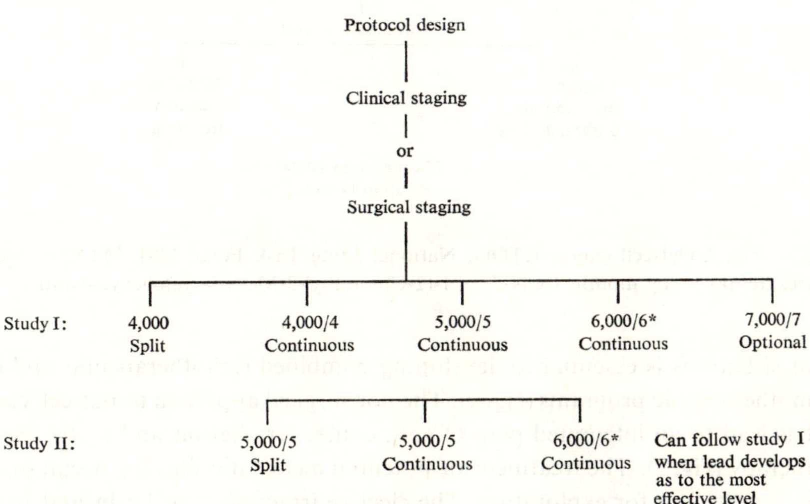

Fig. 2. Lung cancer: squamous cell, adenocarcinoma and large cell undifferentiated - RTOG, National Lung Task Force (29). * = 6,000 rads minimum to T_3, 7,000 rads maximum.

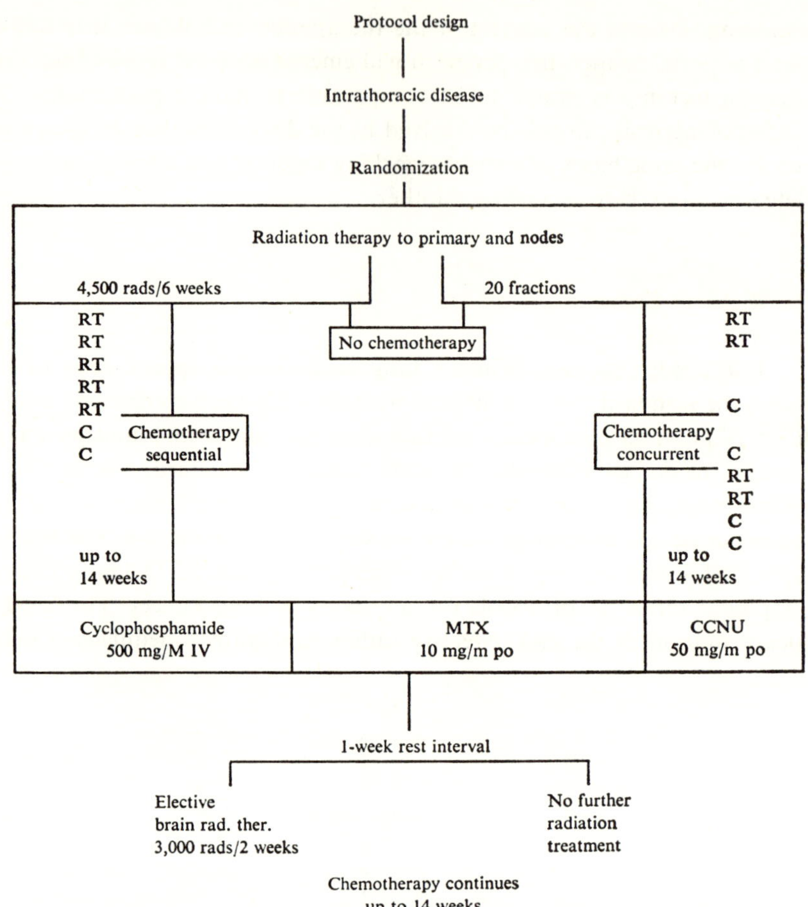

Fig. 3. Oat-cell cancer-RTOG, National Lung Task Force [29]. MTX = Methotrexate, po = by mouth, CCNU = 1-(2-Chlorethyl-3-Methyl-cyclohexyl)-1-nitrosovrea.

of situations is essential to developing combined radiotherapeutic and chemotherapeutic programs (fig. 2). The nonsurgical approach to oat-cell cancer has lead to an integrated plan of split course irradiation and cyclic chemotherapy (fig. 3). The treatment of potential metastatic sites for occult disease is a new area for exploration. The elective irradiation of brain and liver is being considered particularly in oat-cell and other anaplastic cancers. The place of immunotherapy in lung cancers remains undefined; however, there is a large block of patients for study for newer leads in this field.

C. Alimentary Tract

1. Esophagus

For localized stages which are most often intrathoracic and regional-
ized in extent, a standard form of surgical resection is compared to the addition of preoperative irradiation in low to high doses, or the addition of
various chemotherapeutic agents as cyclophosphamide, vincristine, etc.
Advanced and metastatic disease are part of screening phase II drug studies
with single and multiple drugs. In progress at the present time in the RTOG
is the assessment of carbogen breathing with standard doses of irradiation,
i. e., 6,000 rads in 6 weeks. Future studies planned include preoperative irradiation in operable and resectable disease at both low and higher dose
levels, i. e., 2,000–5,000 rads. The purpose of this study is to determine
the optimum dose level to control local disease for unresectable cancers, i. e.,
5,000 rads/4 weeks (Pearson) vs. 6, 000 rads/6 weeks.

2. Stomach

There has been little activity in stomach cancer protocols due to declining
incidence and the poor tolerance of the epigastrium to high doses of irradiation. No protocols are in progress. Some future studies for nonsurgical

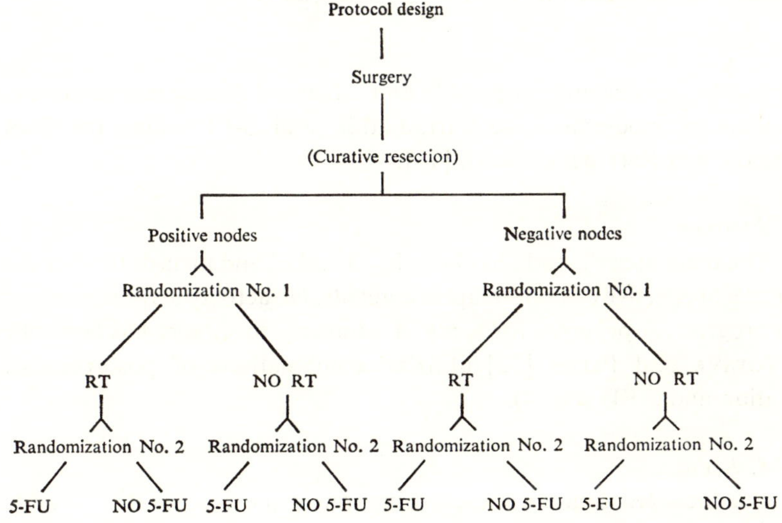

Fig. 4. Clinically eligible patients with Adenocarcinoma of rectum and sigmoid-
RTOG , (32). XRT=000

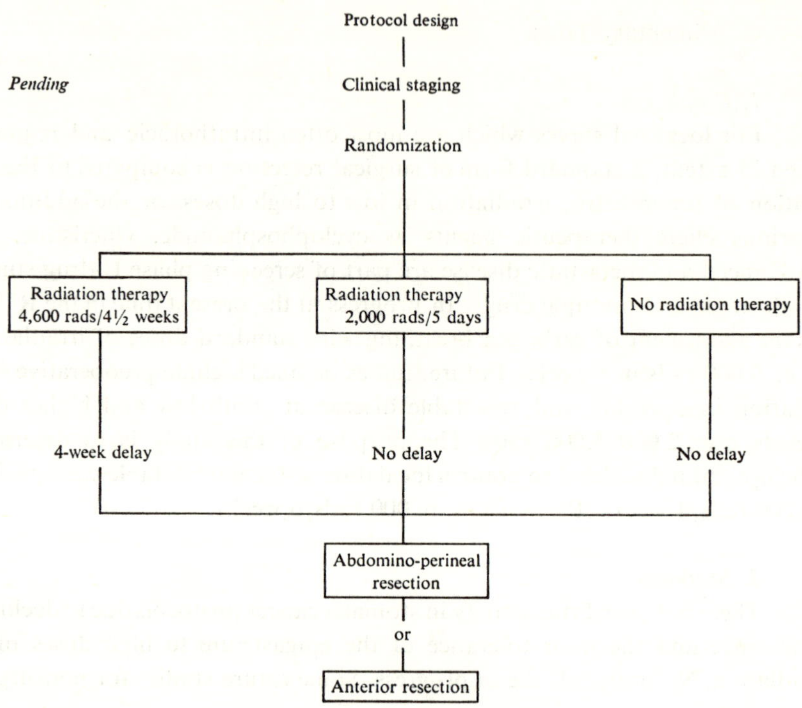

Fig. 5. Rectal cancer - RTOG -Protocol design, COG (14).

approaches in recurrent, inoperable and advanced disease may include combinations of moderate dose x-irradiation and 5-FU along the lines of
MOERTEL and REITMEIER'S work [18].

3. Colon

The main area of study has been in advanced and metastatic liver cancer
in search of effective chemotherapeutic agents. No activity in radiation therapy
is in progress. A proposal for study of adjuvants to surgery has been offered
by VOTAVA and PLENK [32] utilizing combinations of postoperative irradiation and 5-FU (fig. 4).

4. Rectum

For localized cancers, the combination of the preoperative irradiation
and surgery has provoked the most interest and debate. The value of preoperative irradiation can only be resolved by a carefully designed protocol

defining target groups and radiation doses. In progress is a joint protocol offered by KLIGERMAN of the RTOG and GRAGE of the COG [14] in which three options exist: resection alone, low dose-no delay (2,000 rads/5 days) plus resection, and moderate dose-4-week delay (4,000 rads/4½ weeks) plus resection (fig. 5).

D. Female Genital Tract

1. Ovarian Cancer

The major thrust of protocol development has been the exploration of adjuvant procedures with surgical resections. Trials of pre- and post-operative-irradiation, single drugs as thio-tepa and chlorambucil or other alkylation agents have enjoyed most study. The initial development of protocols by the Gynecologic Oncology Group (GOG) chaired by HRESHCHYSHN [12] has been adopted by the RTOG. In stage IA and B ovarian cancer, postoperative irradiation is compared to postoperative chemotherapy (melphelan) as a prophylactic to tumor recurrence (fig. 6). In stage III ovarian cancer, the efficiency of various sequences of radiation therapy and chemotherapy following surgery is being evaluated. Extended fields to include the entire ab-

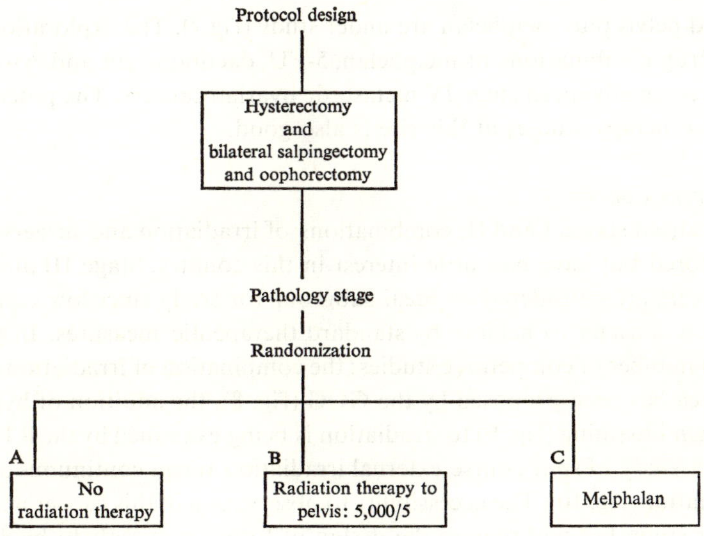

Fig. 6. Ovarian cancer, stages IA and IB - GOG (12).

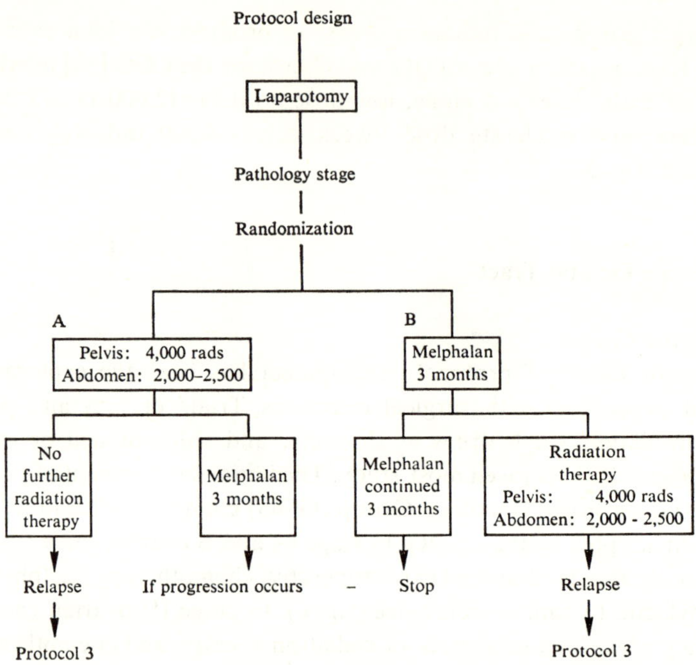

Fig. 7. Ovarian cancer, regionally advanced, stage III - GOG (12).

domen and pelvis plus melphelan are under study (fig.7). The exploration of different drug combinations of melphelan, 5-FU, dactinomycin and cytoxan is in progress in advanced stage IV metastatic ovarian cancers. The potential for immunotherapy studies at this site is also good.

2. Cervix Cancer

In localized stages I and II, combinations of irradiation and surgery are being explored but have had little interest in this country. Stage III and IV cervix cancers are considered an ideal subgroup for study since low control of disease is difficult to achieve by standard therapeutic measures. In progress are a number of competitive studies: the combination of irradiation and hydroxyurea has been proposed by the GOG (fig. 8), the addition of hyperbaric oxygen breathing (fig. 9) to irradiation is being examined by the RTOG as well as a study of split course external irradiation *versus* continuous daily dose irradiation (fig. 10). The accessibility to observation of this cancer makes it ideal for study but will require the design of future protocols to be done with great care and a system of priority.

3. Uterine Fundal Cancers

The value of preoperative irradiation for localized stages has been studied but has not yet been published. The use of progesteron in advanced and recurrent cancers is currently under study. No protocols involving radiation therapy are being planned at present.

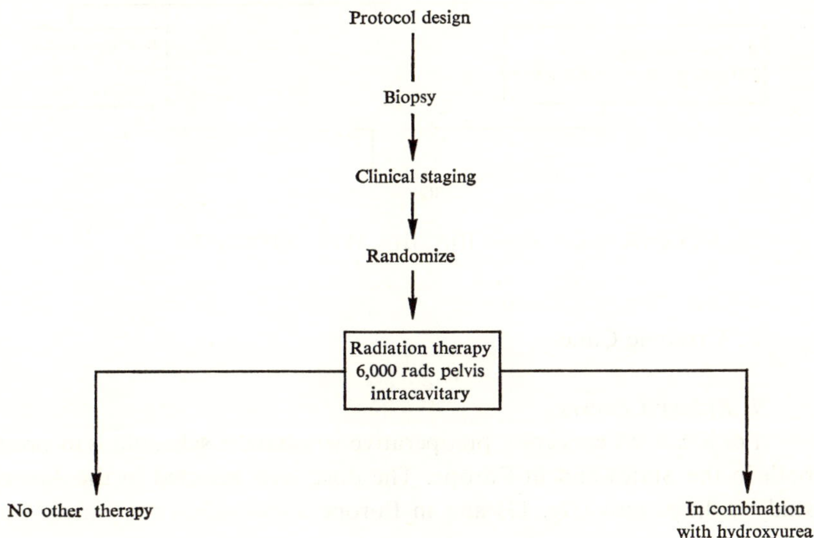

Fig. 8. Cervix cancer, stages III and IV locally advanced - GOG (12).

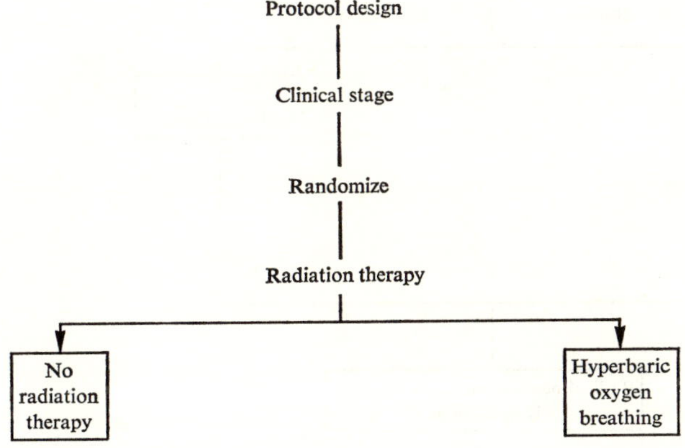

Fig. 9. Cervix cancer, stages IIB, IIIA, IIIB, IVA - RTOG, (3).

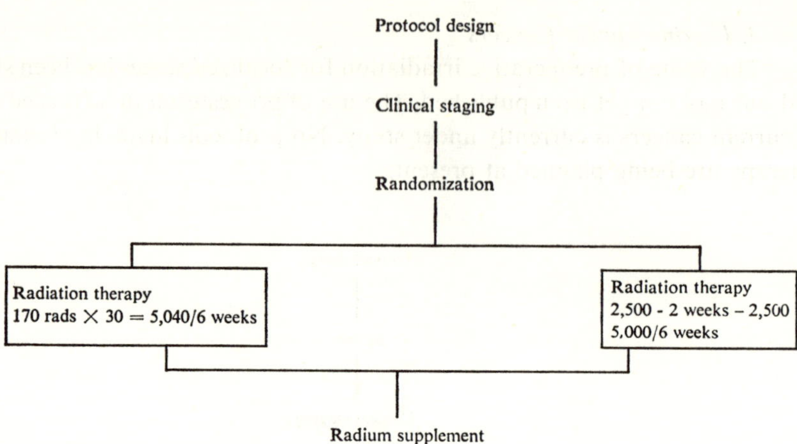

Fig. 10. Cervix cancer, stages IIIA, IIIB, IVA - RTOG (17).

E. Urologic Cancers

1. Kidney Cancers

For localized cancers a preoperative irradiation schedule is in progress both in the States and in Europe. The dose level selected in the American study is 4,500 rads (fig. 11) and in Europe 3,000 rads. In advanced stages,

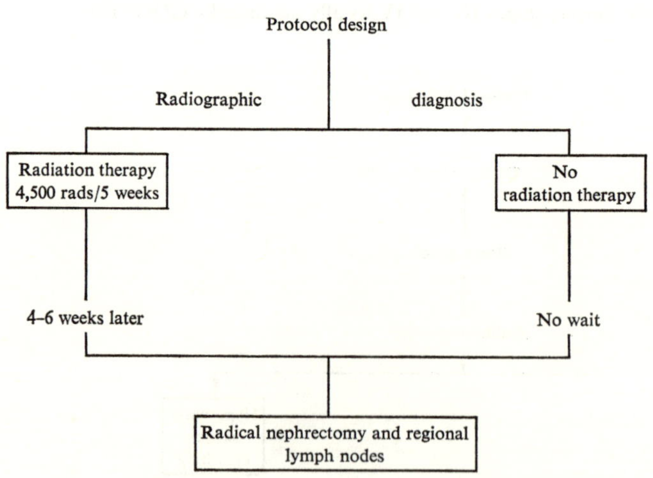

Fig. 11. Renal Cancer, stage: resectable I, II, III - GUOG, (5).

hormonal therapy using progesterone and testosterone as well as chemotherapy are in progress. Future interest in immunotherapy with known patterns of spontaneous remission remains high.

2. Bladder Cancer

For localized stages B and C, there is a lessening of enthusiasm for preoperative irradiation and/or 5-FU based on the poor results in the national study. Renewed interest in comparing curative surgery vs. curative irradiation is being generated by both the GUOG (fig. 12) and the RTOG. An essential new feature of this protocol is staging for pelvic lymph node involvement. In selected cases extended fields for paraortic lymph nodes will be performed if indicated by more elaborate nodal studies. RTOG protocols for hyperbaric oxygen breathing and split course irradiation also exist for bladder cancer in its localized stages B and C.

F. Male Genital Cancers

1. Prostate Cancer

For localized but regionally invasive prostate cancer, stage C, there is DEL REGATO's national protocol (7) comparing irradiation alone vs. irradiation and hormone (fig. 13). For advanced stages, metastatic response to combinations of hormone and/or chemotherapy are being studied by Veterans Administration (VA) hospital groups. The new protocols proposed

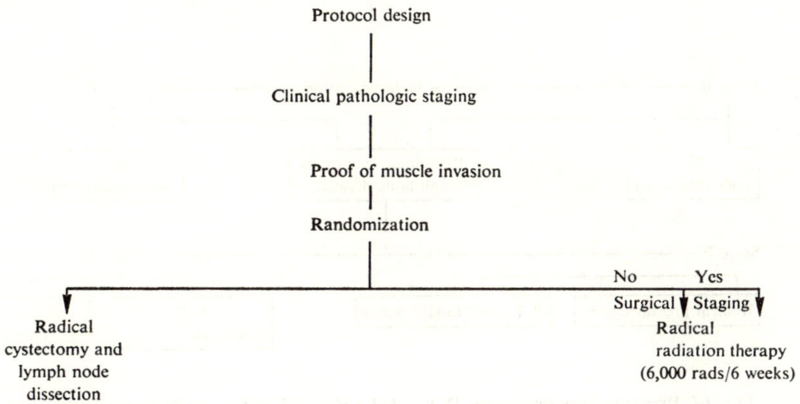

Fig. 12. Bladder cancer, stage B$_2$, C - GUOG, (22).

by the GUOG have been developed by SKINNER [30] for localized stages B and C (fig. 14). The essential new feature is surgical staging with evaluation of lymph nodes by a limited extraperitoneal nodal dissection. In these studies, 7,000 rads axis dose in 47 days to 7,500 rads in 45 days is acceptable range.

2. Testes Cancer

No protocols have emerged of a national nature but an effort to develop a study for nonseminomatous tumors is in progress by the GUOG in collabo-

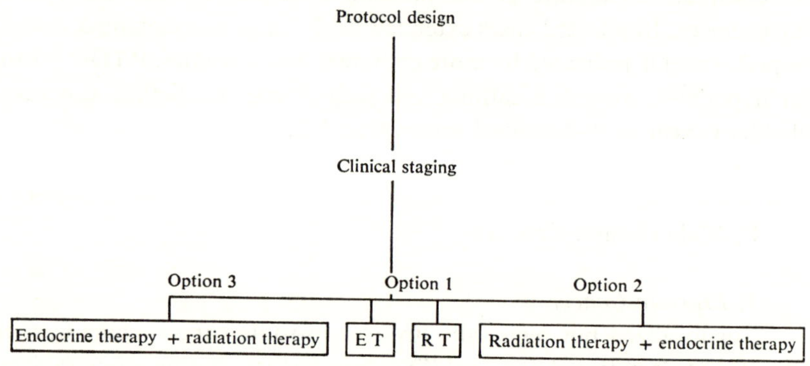

Fig. 13. Prostate cancer, stage C - RTOG (7). ET = endocrine therapy, RT = radiation therapy.

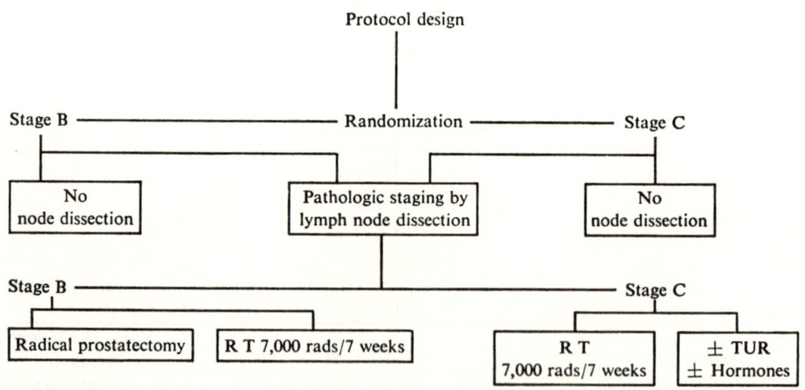

Fig. 14. Prostate cancer, stages B, C – GUOC [30]. RT = radiation therapy, TUR = trans uretheral resection.

ration with other oncology groups. The study will depend on agreement to sequence or alternate retroperitoneal lymphadenectomy, nodal irradiation and chemotherapy for N_0 and N_+ nodes.

G. Head and Neck Cancers

For localized stages without metastatic distant disease, there are numerous protocols combining or comparing surgery and radiation therapy for the primary cancer and neck nodes. A variety of radiation therapy studies evaluating fractionation schedules, combination chemotherapy and irradiation, oxygen breathing at normobaric and hyperbaric conditions exist. In progress are three competing RTOG protocols for oral cavity, oropharynx and hypopharynx cancers of T_3, T_4, N_1, N_2, and N_3 extents. The study of methotrexate combined with irradiation is just being completed with little advantage shown over irradiation alone (fig. 15). In base of tongue and tonsillar cancers, MARCIAL [17] is studying a split course fractional schema vs. continuous course irradiation (figure 16). In a variety of cancers, RUBIN [27] is determining the value of carbogen breathing as an adjuvant to radiation therapy (fig. 17).

Future studies will need to be determined with concern for a system of priority. This is a favored site for assessing tumor control and competitiveness will increase for limited numbers of patients. Combinations of pre- and post-operative irradiation and surgery are being considered. The role of elective

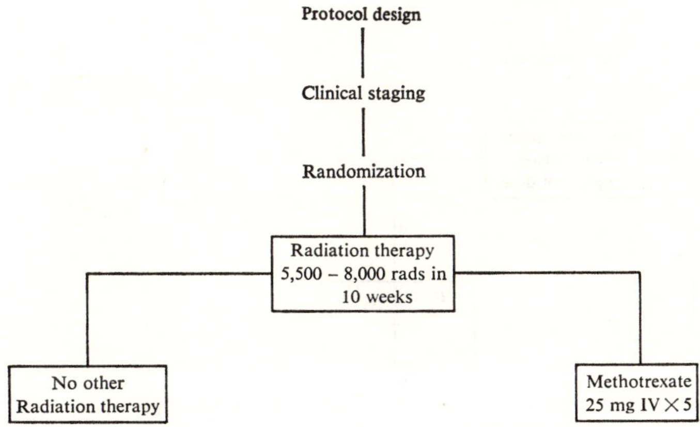

Fig. 15. Oral cavity, oropharynx, hypopharynx - RTOG, (15).

chemotheraphy in advanced cases is being considered based upon responses of different agents in recurrent cases after irradiation and surgery.

H. Central Nervous System (CNS) Tumors

1. Glioblastoma Multiforme

The universal lack of success in controlling the malignant glioma has demanded exploration of nonsurgical approaches. The protocol of the Brain

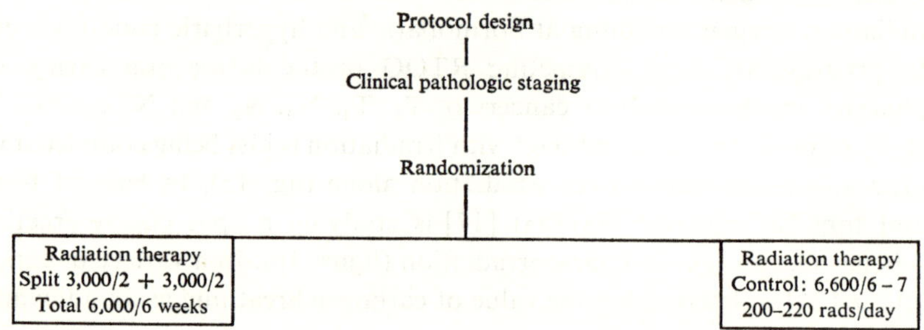

Fig. 16. Base of tongue, tonsillar pillar, all stages - RTOG (17).

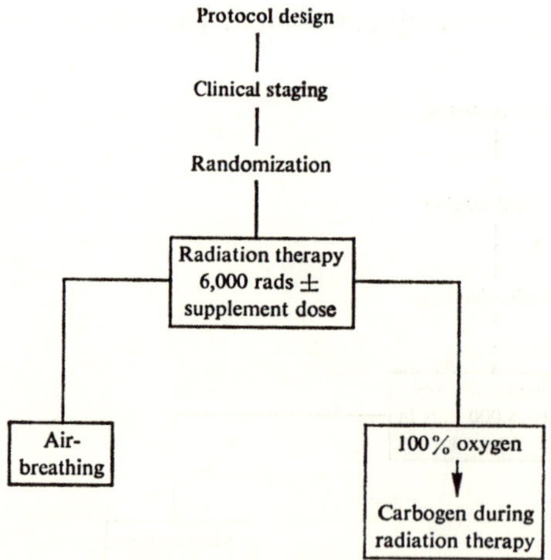

Fig. 17. Oral cavity, hypopharynx, nasopharynx, oropharynx, larynx, esophagus - RTOG (24, 26, 27).

Tumor Surgical Adjuvant Group BTSA chaired by WALKER [33], examined the value of (BCNU) $\pm$ irradiation and found irradiation to be of value in prolonging survival though not effecting cure. A new protocol is being developed jointly by the BTSA and RTOG. Different schedules of irradiation utilizing split course therapy are being considered. Ultra-high doses and combinations of irradiation and multidrugs are under assessment for future study.

2. Metastases

There has been a huge response of cases accessed to the RTOG protocol designed to determine the optimum palliative treatment regimen to maximize the promptness, frequency and duration of symptomatic relief while minimizing morbidity, inconvenience and patient expense. Any patient with known metastatic disease determined by clinical assessment, scans or radiography is acceptable. No primary site is excluded. Five schedules are utilized (fig. 18).

3. Leukemia

The value of elective CNS irradiation in treating sanctuaries of residual cells following chemotherapeutic induction is based upon the observations of AUR et al. [2] at St. Jude's Hospital. Doses up to 2,400 rads to the entire brain and spinal cord are required. Alternate options include: brain irradiation

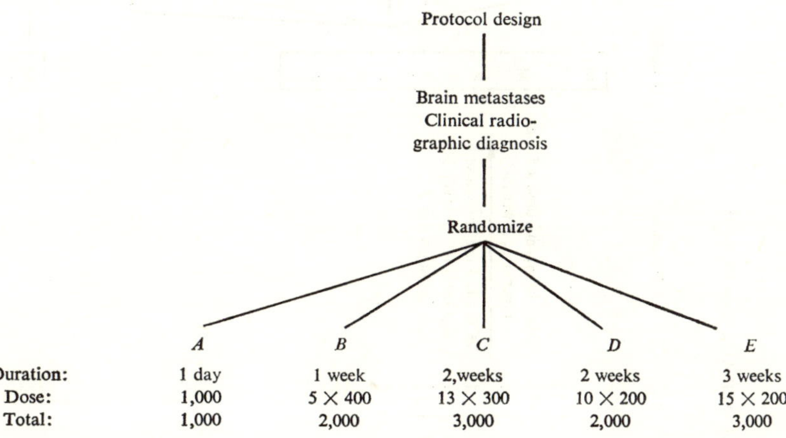

	A	B	C	D	E
Duration:	1 day	1 week	2,weeks	2 weeks	3 weeks
Dose:	1,000	5 × 400	13 × 300	10 × 200	15 × 200
Total:	1,000	2,000	3,000	2,000	3,000

Fig. 18. Brain metastases – RTOG [20]. Steroids are optional but chemotherapy cannot be used.

Schema new ALL/AUL study CCA-101

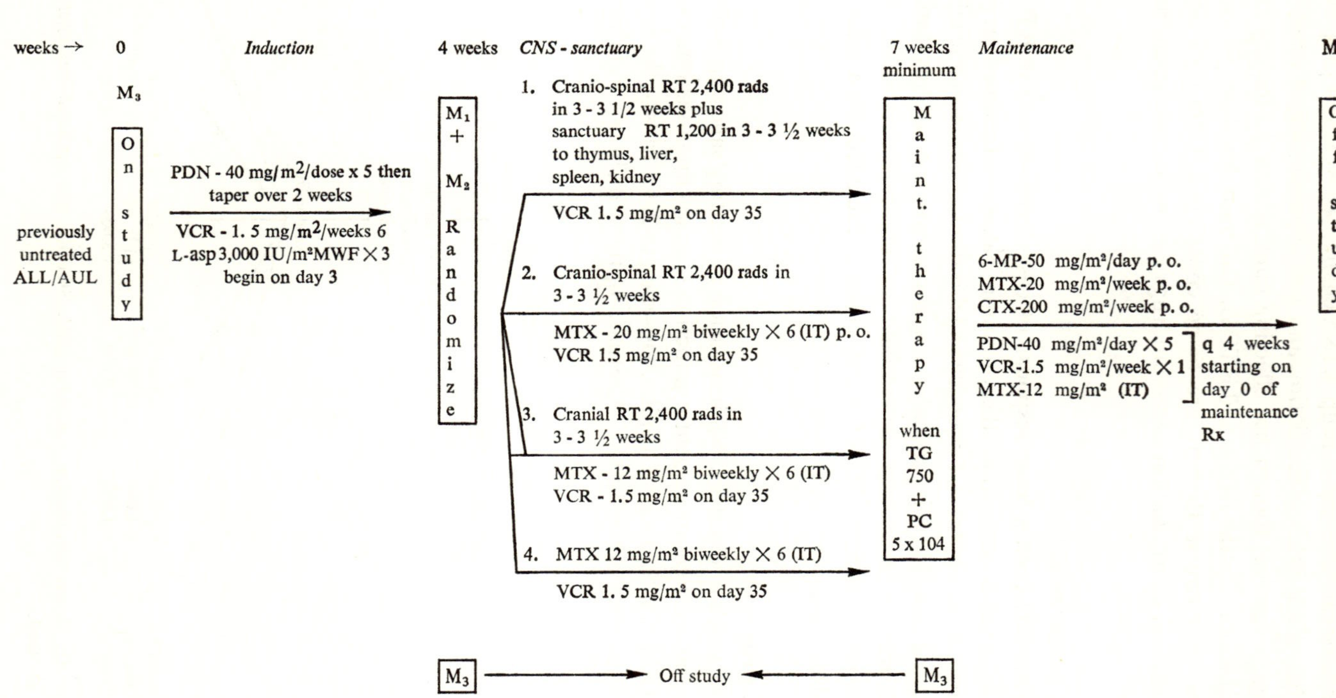

alone; additional elective fields to include: liver, spleen, kidney, thymus plus CNS irradiation; and no irradiation with maintenance chemotherapy (fig. 19). Prednisone, vincristine, and 1-asparginase are employed in obtaining induction in acute lymphocytic leukemia (ALL).

I. Hodgkin's Disease and Lymphomas

1. Hodgkin's disease

The NICKSON and HUTCHINSON [20] protocol exploring the value of extended fields in Hodgkin's disease has confirmed the inability of lymphangiography in excluding the presence of retroperitoneal nodal disease with microscopic foci (fig. 20). The wide use of laparotomy and splenectomy for staging and the introduction of segmental sequential irradiation on both sides of the diaphragm so that nodal treatment is performed has lessened the interest in the outcomes of this study. The European study utilizing vincristine in addition to mantle field irradiation has shown some gain for this combined approach in localized stages I and II with unfavorable histologies as mixed cellularity or lymphocytic depletion. The need for new studies combining multiple drug chemotherapy and extended field irradiation is

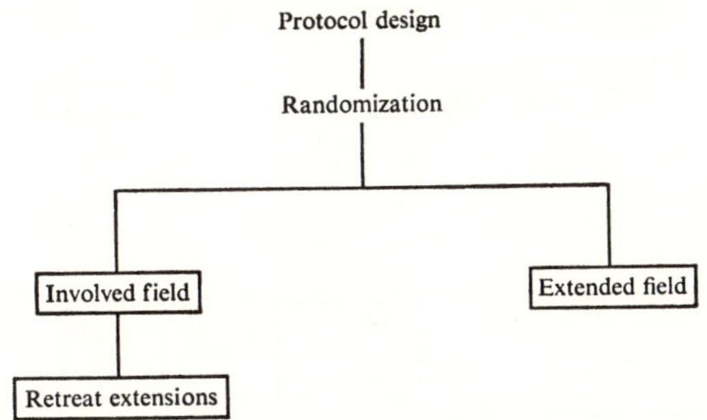

Fig. 20. Hodgkin's disease, stage IA, IIA, IIB - RTOG (20).

Fig. 19. ALL (CNS) – Children's Cancer Study Group A [13]. AUL = Acute undifferentiated leukemia, CCA = Children's Cancer Study Group A, VCR = Vincristine, MTX = Methotrexate, MWF = Monday, Wednesday, Friday, PDN = Prednisone, L-asp = L-asparginase, MP = Mercapto porine, TG = Total granulocytes, PC = Platelet count, IT = intrathecally, p. o. = by mouth, q = every, Rx = Radiation therapy.

apparent. In progress are protocols determining the best sequence of irradiation and multidrug therapy in less favorable stages but in which disease is still confined to the lymph nodes.

2. Lymphomas, Non-Hodgkin's Type

These are protocols studying combinations of drugs to find a sequence of multiple drugs of effectiveness comparable to MOPP in Hodgkin's disease. Such agents as cytoxan, oncovin and prednisone (COP) have been tried with introductions of newer agents as BCNU (fig. 21). The need for an agreement on histopathologic categories is essential to development of target groups for study. In process are emerging protocols modeled along the lines of Hodgkin's disease where segmental sequential irradiation of lymph node regions on both sides of the diaphragm is combined with multidrug therapy. Agreement as to field arrangements, doses of irradiation and combination of drugs needs to be developed.

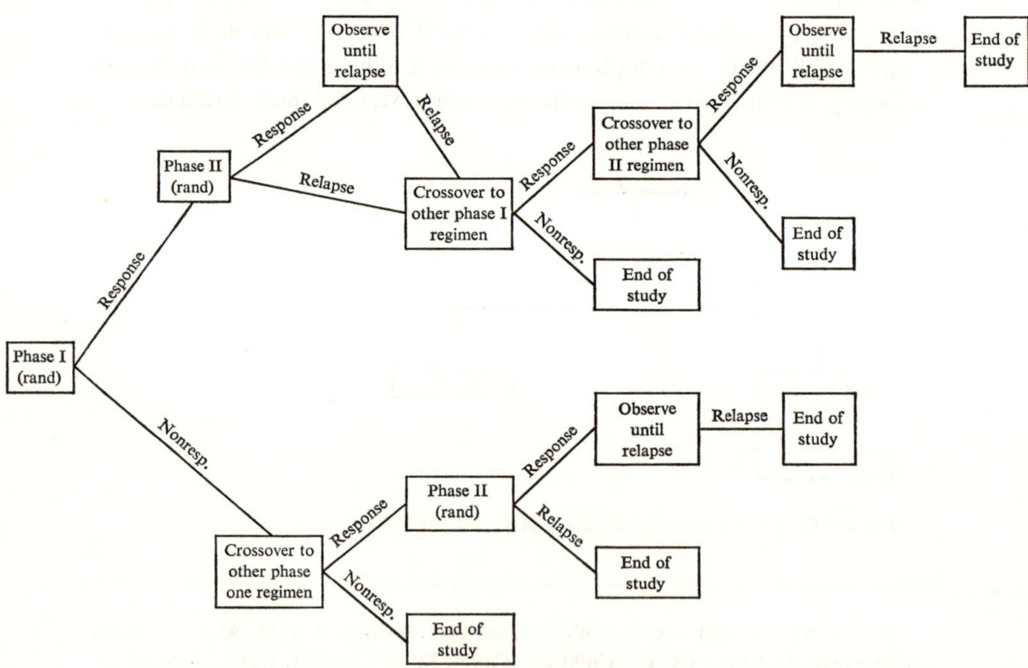

Fig. 21. Intensive *versus* moderate chemotherapy of Lymphosarcoma (lymphocytic lymphoma). Lymphosarcoma, stage III, IV - EST 1472, (19).

J. Pediatric Solid Tumors

1. Wilm's Tumor

The first successful solid tumor study was designed by the National
Wilm's Tumor Study Group. The protocol was based upon the stage of
the disease. The value of postoperative irradiation is being examined in
localized stages and the best combination of chemotherapy in advanced stages
(fig. 22). A failure protocol is an important conceptual design to continue to
accumulate information study in these patients.

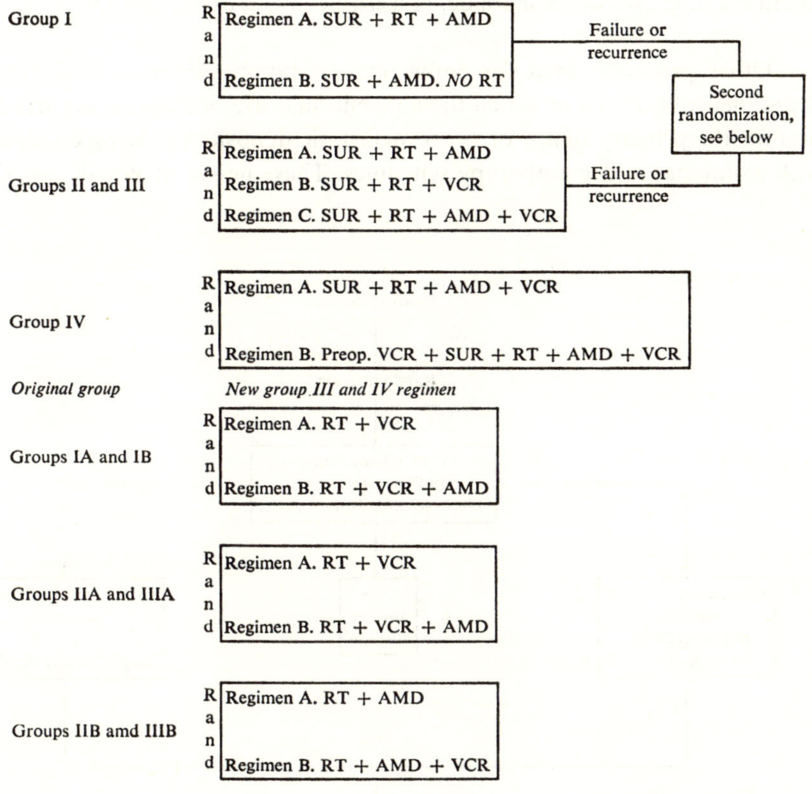

Fig. 22. Wilm's - National Wilm's Tumor Study Group, protocol design. (6).
SUR = surgery, RT = radiotherapy, AMD = actinomycin D, VCR = vincristine.

2. Ewing's Sarcoma

The known high incidence of metastases has lead to the design of a protocol in which primary tumor irradiation 4,000–6,000 rads/4–6 weeks is compared to chemotherapy maintenance (fig. 23).

3. Osteogenic Sarcoma

The protocols developed for osteogenic sarcoma include an elective chemotherapy maintenance program of cyclophosphamide after surgery and/or irradiation. The protocol generated for metastatic disease includes aggressive irradiation of the primary tumor to 6,000 rads/6 weeks, metastatic sites in lung (1,800 rads/2 weeks), liver (3,000 rads) with multiple drug treatment, i. e. cyclophosphamide, vincristine and actinomycin D.

Other protocols exist for embryonal rhabdomysarcoma, histiocytosis X and neuroblastoma in which the conventional use of surgery and irradiation for the primary tumor or overt metastatic deposits are being confirmed with maintenance chemotherapy schedules. These newer protocols are pat-

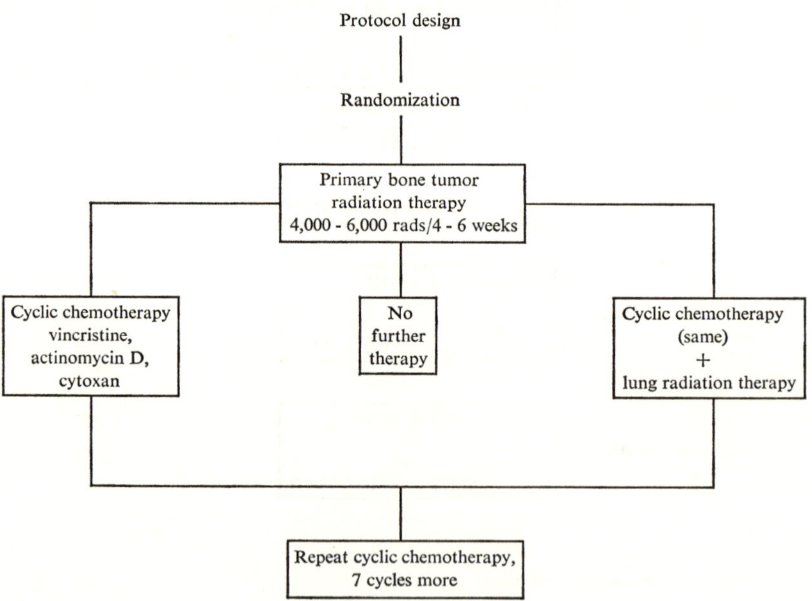

Fig. 23. Bone biopsy, Ewing's sarcoma - Inter-group study, (4).

terned after the Wilm's tumor experience and the more recent success with embryonal rhabdomysarcomas reported from M. D. Anderson Hospital [8].

V. Game and Decision Theory Applied to Establish Priorities

The more complex the decision in medicine, the more often the decision is deferred to the 'experienced' clinician. This is particularly true when the decision is one of 'life and death'. Conflicts of interest invariably develop when specialists consult and offer differing opinions on management. This is a common experience in cancer management; so much so, that tumor boards have been established in many hospitals, to allow for an interface among different disciplines and to encourage a multidisciplinary approach. Conflicts of interest are not unique to medicine; they occur in many different fields and have been a dominant concern of such areas as economics, sociology, political science, etc. The modern mathematical approach to interest conflict, game theory, is credited to VON NEUMANN and MORGENSTERN in their classic book, *Theory of games and economic behavior* [31]. The reason for utilizing this approach is presented in the following evaluation by LUCE and RAIFFA [16].

'It is not difficult to characterize imprecisely the major aspects of the problem of interest conflict: an individual is in a situation from which one of several possible outcomes will result and with respect to which he has certain personal preferences. However, though he may have some control over the variables which determine the outcome, he does not have full control. Sometimes this is in the hands of several individuals who, like him, have preferences among the possible outcomes, but who in general do not agree in their preferences. In other cases, chance events (which are sometimes known in law as 'acts of God') as well as other individuals (who may or may not be affected by the outcome of the situation) may influence the final outcome. The types of behavior which result from such situations have long been observed and recorded, and it is a challenge to devise theories to explain the observations and to formulate principles to guide intelligent action.'

Game theory does not, and probably no mathematical theory could, encompass all of the diverse problems of medicine which are characterized by conflicts of interest. Let us, however, explore this approach in cancer management. Firstly, it is assumed with respect to the general choices of surgery, radiotherapy and chemotherapy that each specialist physician has a consistent pattern of preferences: it is further supposed that if he were offered a collection of alternatives, his choice could be ascertained under a variety of conditions. Secondly, the variables which control possible outcomes are assumed to be well specified. Conflicts of interest arise when there are a number of clinicians, each of whom is required to make one choice from a well defined set of possible choices, often without knowledge as to the choices of other clinicians. Game theory deals with the choices that players, in this case clinicians, may make; or rather with the choices that they *should* make, in their attempt to improve the outcomes of treatments.

Cancer decision-making can be done by an individual clinician or by a multidisciplinary group, whether it is effected under conditions of (1) certainty; (2) risk, or (3) uncertainty. In game theory, the certainty-risk-uncertainty classification in choosing between two alternatives is made according to the following conditions:

1. *Certainty* if each action is known to lead invariably to a specific outcome.

2. *Risk* if each action leads to one of a set of possible outcomes, each occurring with known probability.

3. *Uncertainty* if each action has a set of specific outcomes, but where the probabilities of the outcomes are completely unknown.

Many mathematical formulations have been made with regard to individual and even group decision-making under these conditions. In his book entitled *Social choice and individual values* (1), ARROW attempts to resolve the problem of how best to amalgamate the discordant preference patterns of a group and arrive at a compromise. To achieve such a result, modern utility theory is used as a cornerstone of decision theory; for the cancer specialist, this can be viewed as the equivalent of a long-term survival free of disease and complications of treatment.

The game of GOPS (*game of pure strategy*) [16] which is based upon card games, lends itself to analysis by construction of game trees. Such a game tree for a three-handed card game can be used as a model for cancer decision making (fig. 24). For each cancer patient, there are three major decision points related to surgery, radiation therapy and chemotherapy. Each clinician has three choices, but can make only one move. The sequence of moves and choices, one following the other, is the preferred treatment plan (in game theory-play). Plan (or play) means a detailed statement of the actual decisions made. A decision tree of therapeutic stratagems allows the clinician to recognize his options. Such a frame is essential for the formulation of cooperative studies and multidisciplinary protocols.

Since the choice of any two options blocks the utilization of the other 30-some alternatives that are theoretically possible, an order of preference

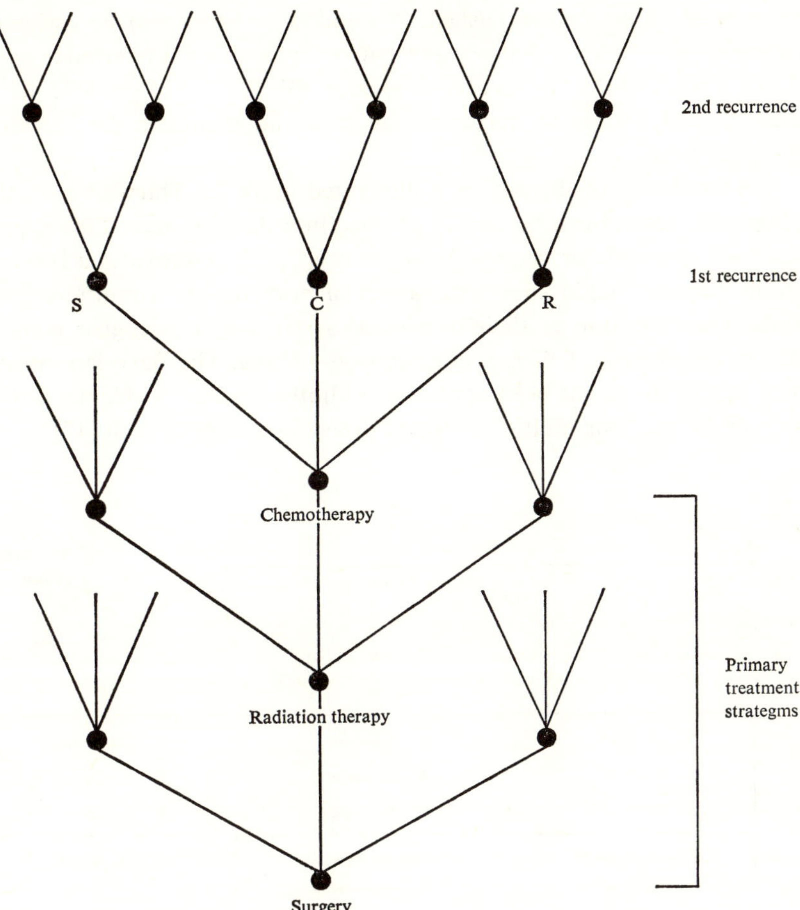

Fig. 24. Game and decision theory. Game of GOPS: decision tree. The 'game of GOPS' refers to *game of pure strategy*. The model for this is a 3-handed card game, in which there is one winner. This game can be applied to cancer management problems, when seen from a multidisciplinary point of view. For each cancer patient there are 3 players: surgeon (S), radiotherapist (R) and chemotherapist (C). Each has a primary decision to make; if an option is not exercised, all this means is that the decision was made not to exercise it. Unidisciplinary decision, therefore, has been substituted for what could have been multidisciplinary decision. When a choice is made for a cancer patient, there are always 30-35 other options which could have been exercised, but were not. This is the way in which one can view the multidisciplinary decision-making process (31).

or priorities must be established. A number or index can be assigned to basic alternatives, such that one alternative (or gamble) is preferred to another if its expected utility (or success) is greater. Given a set of possible acts, the clinician will choose to maximize the gain and minimize the loss due to complications.

A tabulation of alternatives is illustrated in fig. 25. Thirty or more therapeutic alternatives can be viewed at once in a decision tree. This approach has been detailed for genito-urinary cancers [15]. It provides a format for group decision-making and assignment of priorities on a multidisciplinary basis. The definition of their own value systems by oncologists is another step in the process of therapeutic decision-making. The Bayesian model for such deliberations has been applied to radiotherapeutic problems; however, it could be used for multidisciplinary decision-making as well [17].

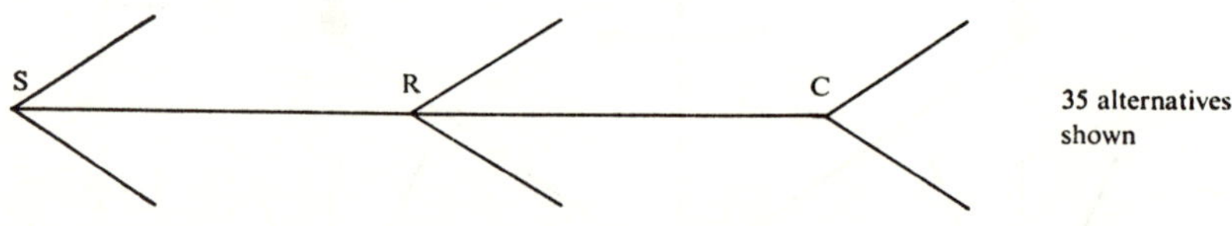

S Standard	R Standard	C Single drug
S Extended	R Extended	C Multiple drugs
S Decreased	R Decreased	C Cyclic
S ⟶ R	R ⟶ S	C vs. R vs. S
R ⟶ S	S ⟶ R	
RS	RS	C + R + S
R ⟶ S ⟶ R	R ⟶ S ⟶ R	C ⟶ R ⟶ S
S ⟶ R ⟶ S	S ⟶ R ⟶ S	C ⟶ S ⟶ R
		R ⟶ C ⟶ S
C ⟶ S	C ⟶ R	R ⟶ S ⟶ C
S ⟶ C	R ⟶ C	S ⟶ R ⟶ C
CS	RC	S ⟶ C ⟶ R
C ⟶ S ⟶ C	C ⟶ R ⟶ C	

Fig. 25. Cancer treatment options. The game of GOPS model shows 3 alternatives in cancer management: surgery (S), radiation therapy (R) and chemotherapy (C). If standard form of treatment is accepted, there are two possibilities. For each modality they can be extended (made more radical) or decreased (made more conservative). The tabulation below the model indicates at least 35 alternatives or combinations of treatment.

The rational basis for cooperative clinical studies in radiation therapy and oncology has been presented above. A review of ongoing trials in the United States has been summarized, and a brief statement of their purpose and progress has been provided. The RTOG was constituted for the express purpose of conducting and organizing clinical studies in the United States. The 'game of GOPS' has been applied as a model for multidisciplinary decision-making in cancer studies, and as such is highly recommended.

References

1   Arrow, K. J.: Social choice and individual values, 2nd ed. (Wiley, New York 1963).
2   Aur, R. J. A.; Simone, J.; Hustu, H. O.; Walters, T.; Borella, L.; Pratt, C., and Pinkel, D.: Central nervous system therapy and combination chemotherapy of childhood lymphocytic leukemia. Blood, *37*:272–281 (1971).
3   Brady, L.: Hyperbaric oxygen protocol. Radiation Therapy Oncology Group (1972).
4   Burgert, O.; Nesbit, M. E.; Vietti, T.; Gehan, E.; Ackerman, L. V.; Childs, D., and Griffen, P.: National Ewing's sarcoma study. Clinical trial of combined surgery, radiotherapy and chemotherapy in previously untreated Ewing's sarcoma. Inter-Group Study (1970).
5   Cox, C.E.: Renal cell carcinoma study. Radiotherapy, intercalibration of radio-therapeutic sources. Genito-Urinary Oncology Group (1969).
6   D'Angio, G.: Children with Wilm's tumor. Wilm's Tumor Study Group (1970).
7   Regato, J. Del: Radiotherapy in the conservative treatment of operable and locally inoperable carcinoma of the prostate. Rad. *88*:761–766, (1967).
8   Donaldson, S. S.; Castro, J. R.; Wilbur, J. R., and Jesse, R. H., jr.: Rhabdomyos-arcoma of head and neck in children: Combination treatment by surgery, irradiation and chemotherapy. Cancer *31*:26–35 (1973).
9   Ezdinli, E. Z.; Brunk, S. F., and Aungst, W.: Evaluation of intensive versus moderate chemotherapy in lymphosarcoma (lymphocytic lymphoma). Eastern Cooperative Oncology Group (1972).
10   Fisher, B.: Postoperative radiotherapy in the treatment of breast cancer: Results of the NSABP clinical trial. Ann. Surg. *172*:711–732 (1970).
11   Flamant, R. (ed.): Controlled therapeutic trials in cancer. UICC Technical Report Series, vol. 8 (Union Internationale Contre le Cancer, Geneva 1972).
12   Hreshchyshn, M. M.: Protocols for ovarian cancer and cervix cancer. Submitted to the Radiation Therapy Oncology Group (1972).
13   Klemperer, M.: Treatment of newly diagnosed acute lymphocytic/undifferentiated leukemia with intensive chemotherapy and radiotherapy. Children's Cancer Study Group A (1972).
14   Kligerman, M. and Grage, T. B.: Protocol for rectal cancer. Submitted to the Radiation Therapy Oncology Group (1972).

15 KRAMER, S.: Protocol for the controlled study to determine the value of combined irradiation and chemotherapy for squamous cell carcinoma of the oral cavity, pharynx and larynx. Radiation Therapy Oncology Group (1969).

16 LUCE, R. D. and RAIFFA, H.: Games and decisions: Introduction and critical survey. (Wiley, New York 1957).

17 MARCIAL, V.: Newly developed split course radiation therapy protocol. Submitted to the Radiation Therapy Oncology Group (1970).

18 MOERTEL, C. G. and REITMEIER, R. J.: Advanced gastro-intestinal cancer: Clinical management and chemotherapy (Harper & Row, New York 1967).

19 MUSTAKILLIO, S.: Treatment of breast cancer by tumor extirpation and roentgen therapy instead of radical operation. Clin. Rad. *6*:23–26 (1954).

20 NICKSON, J. J. and HUTCHINSON, G. B.: Hodgkin's disease clinical trials. Proc. Nat. Cancer Conf. *6*:77–81 (1970).

21 PETERS, M. V.: Wedge resection and irradiation. J. Amer. Med. Assoc. *200*:2 (1967).

22 PROUT, G. R.; SLACK, N. H., and BROSS, I. D. J.: Preoperative irradiation as an adjuvant in the surgical management of invasive carcinoma. J. Urol. *105*:223–231 (1971).

23 RIGBY-JONES, P.: The influence of various factors on matastases in carcinoma of the breast. Brit. J. Cancer *7*:431–437 (1953).

24 RUBIN, P.: Current concepts in genito-urinary oncology: A multidisciplinary approach. J. Urol. *106*:315–338 (1971).

25 RUBIN, P. (ed.): Investigative therapeutics in clinical oncology (University of Rochester Press, Rochester 1972).

26 RUBIN, P.: Discussion: The choice and meaning of tolerance in radiotherapeutics: The Bayesian model; in Vaeth, Front. Radiation Ther. Onc., vol. 6 (Karger, Basel, and University Park Press, Baltimore 1972).

27 RUBIN, P.: Protocol for carbogen-oxygen breathing. Radiation Therapy Oncology Group (1971).

28 SCHOTZ, W. E.: Protocol for palliation of symptomatic osseous and brain metastases. Radiation Therapy Oncology Group (1971).

29 SELAWRY, O.: Clinical trials of cancer of the lung. Submitted to the Radiation Therapy Oncology Group (1972).

30 SKINNER, D.: Prostate cancer stages B and C Protocol. Submitted to the Genito-Urinary Oncology Group (1972).

31 NEUMANN, J. VON and MORGENSTERN, O.: Theory of games and economic behavior, 3rd. ed. (Princeton University Press, Princeton 1953).

32 VOTAVA, C., jr. and PLENK, H. P.: A controlled pilot study to determine the value of post-operative irradiation and 5-FU as adjuvant therapy to surgery in the treatment of colorectal carcinomas. Submitted to the Radiation Therapy Oncology Group (1972).

33 WALKER, E.: Protocol for glioblastoma multiforme. Submitted to the Brain Tumor Surgical Adjuvant Group (1970).

Author's address: Dr. PHILIP RUBIN, Division of Therapeutic Radiology, Strong Memorial Hospital, University of Rochester, *Rochester, NY 14520* (USA)

Front. Radiation Ther. Onc., vol. 8, pp. 175–185
(Karger, Basel and University Park Press, Baltimore 1973)

Data Recall, Clinical Research and the Cancer Center[1]

T. L. PHILLIPS

Section of Radiation Oncology, University of California, San Francisco, Calif.

Introduction

For many years, clinicians and clinical investigators have recognized the importance of the collection of medical data. A reasonably standardized form of data collection, the patient chart or medical record, has evolved. It is now evident that this classical record is not adequate for the needs of either the cancer center or, indeed, of general medical institutions [1]. Both WEED [7, 8] and HURST [2, 3] have pointed out the failure of present medical record systems to properly organize data, identify problems, solve problems and teach students. WEED has devised a new problem-oriented approach to the medical record and is now applying this approach to the development of a computerized medical record system.

In addition to the basic needs of a cancer center and, indeed, any medical center, to organize data, solve problems and teach, there is an even greater duty to analyze the results of conventional and experimental treatment. As OSLER said [4]: 'If you have the good fortune to command a large clinic, remember that one of your chief duties is tabulation and analysis of the carefully recorded experience.' This admonition is particularly true for those in charge of a cancer center, oncology service or radiation therapy department.

1   This work was support in part by the Area I Regional Cancer Program of the California Committee for Regional Medical Programs.

Failures in the Present Data Recall Systems

The present format of medical record-keeping is source-oriented, disorganized, and exists only in a single or sometimes duplicate copy (as in radiotherapy departments). Such records are not amenable to rapid analysis. Each time the experience in treating 30 cases of a rather rare tumor or 500 cases of a common tumor is to be reviewed it becomes a major project, usually only carried out with publication in mind. Often, a resident is assigned to review the cases and a staff physician supervises and reviews his review. Since the records are not problem-oriented and do not have a fixed format data base, they do not contain a predefined amount of information – an important factor is often missing. These reviews, once published, become the gospel for future treatment in spite of the very limited and dated nature of the results.

Clinical decisions are usually made on the basis of reports in the literature gathered as described above or even more often based on remembered cases, a spotty and faulty memory at best. It is not possible to review a significant number of patients, their response to treatment, and then select the most successful treatment because the only tool available is a cross-index of cases and the voluminous paper chart which must be individually read.

The conventional tumor registry, although having served a need and collected a limited number of data on a large amount of patients, has not met the requirements for availability of data in making clinical judgments. The data stored in such registries is limited to a few broad categories and is extremely limited in its description of the extent of disease and details of therapy. Many of the registries are not computerized and very few are accessible on real time remote terminals.

Data Recall and the Cancer Center

When a decision has been made to improve the care of patients with cancer through the formation of a cancer center within an institution, city or region, the inclusion of suitable data recording and recall systems must be planned as part of the center design. If the best and most modern care is to be offered to patients attending the center, the physicians in the center must know the result of treatment of different types for each cancer site, histology and extent of disease prior to choosing therapy for a new patient.

It is imperative to have available the updated results of one's own experience and specific treatment techniques as well as those of the region and eventually of the nation for comparison.

If the requirements for an operational data system as a portion of the cancer center are accepted, then it is obvious that the center must work toward an entirely new patient-record system which is designed for rapid retrieval and for the correlation of information stored within the system. This system should be readily available at all times and be updated on a day-to-day basis. It should evolve towards the complete replacement of the conventional medical records and the conventional tumor registry.

Clinical Trials within a Cancer Center

One of the major functions of an institutional or regional cancer center will be in conducting clinical trials of new treatment regimes at various levels. The proper evaluation of response of patients in such trials requires recording of a specific uniform data base for each entered patient, the organization of the data and the frequent review of the results. In some cases, these trials will be national and controlled from a central office. This does not obviate the need for the individual center to know the results in patients who have entered into such trials. At the present time, almost every new national trial has designed for it a set of unfamiliar complex and confusing paper data forms. Since the basic data set for all cancer cases is similar and since the only major difference is the description of the site of involvement, it would seem highly desirable to evolve a standard data base for clinical trials within an institution and on a national basis. The current system also creates a triple duplication of effort. One is creating a conventional medical record, a local registry of some type and the forms for the national trial. It should be possible to combine all of these efforts into one computerized medical record. The present system, in addition to its expense and additional effort, often leads to the situation in which the results of national trials are not available for months or years and are often outdated when finally published.

The goals for planning for data handling in a cancer center should be the solution of this problem by the establishment of a uniform data base, method of recording, and method of retrieval which is compatible with the desires of national groups.

Data Recall Systems Available for Oncology

There are approximately 6 major types of data storage and retrieval systems available. These are outlined in table I and include systems which range from the simplest disease-specific index card system which lists the names of patients with a specific code number or site of disease up to a completely automated computerized storage and retrieval system as being developed at the University of Vermont by WEED [8] and by SCHULTZ *et al.* [6]. Although the first 4 types of systems are quite simple and easily understood, it may be of use to describe in somewhat more detail the computer-stored detailed data base developed by us in the Area 1 California Regional Medical Programs [5] and the completely automated problem-oriented record system development by WEED and colleagues [8].

The California Regional Medical Program Area 1 Cancer Data Retrieval System has been described in detail by PHILLIPS *et al.* [5]. It is disease-oriented, rather than patient-oriented, and is concerned with one class of disease–cancer. The primary emphasis in system design has been physician accessibility. The entry system in use is an auxiliary paper form input based on a basic data set consisting of 7 different sets of paper forms designed for key punch input (table II). The identification section includes such items as marital status, race, level of activity and major occupation, which make up the basic patient profile. The next major portion of the data base is the record

Table I. Data recall systems for oncology

Disease-specific index cards – conventional records
Mechanical cross-index systems – conventional records
Hole-pin
Termatrex
Computer-stored cross-indices – key punched input
Computer-stored minimum data base – key punched input
Name, age, sex, diagnosis, dose of radiation, etc.
Computer-stored detailed data base – key punched input
Problems, extent of disease, treatment details, follow-up
May provide some portions of conventional record
Complete automatic computer-stored system – CRT input
Question trees on CRT terminals
Automatic input of laboratory treatment data
Completely replaces conventional record
CRT output at numerous stations
Eventually integrated into institutional system

Table II. Basic data set – (RMP) – DRS

---

1. Identification – patient profile
2. Diagnosis – problem list
3. Extent of disease, symptoms, site-specific
4. Radiotherapy summary – external, brachytherapy
5. Chemotherapy summary – initial and final
6. Surgery summary
7. Progress note – follow-up

---

of diagnosis and important associated problems. A diagnosis record and problem list also includes the evaluation of the patient's functional status, his social history of alcoholism, etc., and the family history of cancer.

The third and most detailed section of the data base is the extent of disease record. There are 39 individual formats which cover the major anatomic sites of disease as well as specific entities such as lymphomas, soft tissue sarcomas, and benign, non-neoplastic, disease. These forms include detailed questions as to the status of the primary tumor, the direct extension of the tumor, the regional lymph nodes and the distant metastases. They also include evaluation of specific signs and symptoms relative to the particular sites.

The next section of the record is the radiotherapy summary which includes both external beam and brachytherapy forms. They include sufficient detail to evaluate treatment energy, field size and location, numbers of fractions and other information recorded for formulas such as that used for the calculation of NSD. The chemotherapy summary is divided into an initial summary filled out after 2 months and a final summary when the specific drugs administered are discontinued. The forms include the definition of measurable parameters, the functional status of the patient prior to therapy, the specific agent used and the response of the patient to treatment. The surgery summary is designed in a general format which allows evaluation of the extent of removal of the primary organ, the primary tumor and the regional lymphatics, as well as the nature of any residual tumor following surgery and any complications of wound-healing or surgical problems.

The final form is a detailed evaluation of the patient's progress at each evaluation for follow-up. It includes the patient's symptomatology, and the objective findings of tumor involvement in primary, regional or metastatic sites and any planned future treatment. The follow-up information is added 3, 6 and 12 months after treatment and thereafter every 6 months.

A primary goal in the design of the system was ready access on a real time basis using a remote computer terminal. The retrieval system designed is basically a browsing system. One important consideration in designing the system was accessibility to physicians regardless of former computer experience. The records are organized and filed on computer discs by site of disease. Because of the disc file rapid access system, limits are placed on the size of each section and each record has a fixed format.

The remote processing system currently available at the University of California San Francisco is the IBM conversational program system (CPS). The specific programming knowledge required is limited to the small details of logging-in and logging-out as well as loading the browsing system program. At the present time, there is a total of 10 functions available on the remote browsing system. These are shown in table III. The first three functions, data base, subset and merge, are used to create the population and subpopulation which one wishes to study or to compare with other populations. This population may then be used to obtain numbers of patients with specific individual criteria from the more than 1,500 bits of information or may be used to generate survival rates, correlations, staging information or distributions of numerical values. Individual variables may be listed on a remote terminal or requested for rapid batch listing on the line printer located at the computer center.

This system has led to the design of a specific data base which seems quite relevant after the entry of 3,000 cases into the system over the past year. It has the major drawback of requiring duplicate information entry

Table III. RMP-DRS browsing system

Functions
1. Data base
2. Subset
3. Merge
4. Survival rate
5. Correlation
6. Staging and survival
7. Distribution
8. List variables
9. Batch list
10. Hard copy-data base summary

since it at present does not replace any part of the medical records. Although dedicated physicians have been able to enter data, it does require careful checking by trained data technologists prior to entry into the computer. The feedback into the system is slow and the remote terminal operation using the IBM CPS is also relatively slow. It is clear, in order to make this a permanently valuable system, that it must be transformed into an automatic entry system which can replace the cumbersome dictating of patient histories, replace the present hard copy medical record with an automatically printed record and, at the same time, automatically enter data into disc files in a retrievable format.

The other system, which is now in use at the University of Vermont, is a problem-oriented medical record adapted for remote cathode ray tube (CRT) terminal input and display using an interactive terminal and a human interface program [6]. In this system, computer terminals are used for the retrieval of patient records and paper copies are only kept for back-up purposes and the final hospital record. The system is based on a philosophy requiring the medical data to be organized in a problem-oriented fashion rather than a source-oriented fashion. The data are collected, filed and stored with respect to a specific problem among the several problems shown by the patient and not according to the source of data. Since the problem oriented medical record as derived by WEED [7] requires a systematic approach to treatment, this approach is defined by the 4 phases of medical action, i.e.: data base collection, problem formulation, definition of the treatment plan and follow-up patient response. These basic 4 phases of medical action, as described by WEED [7, 8] and developed by HURST and WALKER [3] are outlined in table IV. After the initial data base collection, each phase of medical action is related to each specific problem. In other words, the plans, progress notes, orders and discharge summaries are listed separately for each problem as defined in the complete problem list. In the hands of WEED and HURST this system has proven to be an excellent educational tool and a better method or organizing medical data for evaluation and for teaching. It has also proved to be an excellent way of organizing data for computer storage and recall, since each plan and order and each progress note may be oriented to specific initial problems. Information stored may be related to each problem, thus making retrieval program design simplier.

In order to directly interface medical personnel to the computer system, the group at Vermont used a remote CRT terminal on which a display of choices is made. The user chooses one or many of these offered choices by simply touching an indicated section of the screen with his finger. The user

Table IV. The problem-oriented record

Data base
      Patient profile
      History
      Physical
      Laboratory
      Radiologic

Complete problem list
      1
      2
      3
      4

Initial plans
      1. First problem   2. Second problem, etc.
      Diagnostic
      Therapeutic
      Patient education

Progress notes

      Narrative notes
      1. First problem   2. Second problem, etc.
      Subjective
      Objective
      Assessment
      Plans
      Flow sheet
      Discharge summary

---

selection is put into the system as a form of character for each of the 20 available positions on the screen. Following a initial selection, appropriate branching takes place and new questions or information are displayed on the screen. The basic data base collection is done by a large series of frames on displays designed for questioning or branching as indicated by the initial response.

The selections made by the user from the frames at the terminal are organized by the human interface program to form a paragraph of recorded information. These paragraphs are the basic unit of information generated in the system. The user-generated paragraph and the associated selection parameter list related to frame number and choice within the frame are the mechanisms which couple the human interface program and the application program which store, retrieve and manipulate the records.

Because the system has been designed for general medical use in all phases of medicine, the collection of the original data base and the development of plans and progress notes must be broad. Thus, there are currently over 16,000 possible screen displays in the system. Approximately 12,000 of these are branching displays.

This system is currently oriented toward the individual patient record in its storage format and has not been oriented toward mass retrieval across many patient records. However, the compact nature of the storage in conjunction with limitations on the size of the data base could readily convert it into a rapid retrieval system for analyzing multiple records as well as for analyzing an individual record.

Achieving the Optimum Data System within the Cancer Center

As discussed above, the cancer center will not be able to meet its goals of optimum patient care, demonstration and clinical research without entirely new systems of computer-stored and recallable records. The ultimate design of such a system is complex and has not yet been accomplished in any single institution, let alone in a cancer center. The eventual goal can be approached from three directions. Some initial compromises will be necessary in order to allow continued efficient operation of the existing cancer services and centers while the optimum data, storage, and recall system is developed within the institution and within the nation.

Common to all three approaches to the problem is the formulation of a minimum oncology data base which includes subjective, objective, summary and follow-up data required for all cancer patients. This minimum data base must contain the portions of the patient profile, history, physical and laboratory data which are relevant to the problems of cancer. It must include those portions of the problem list which in any way relate to the patient's cancer and its prognosis as well as the plan and summary of treatment and the evaluation of the patient's progress through detailed follow-up notes. If such a data base is properly designed, and collected with the input of oncologists across the country and from the disciplines of surgical, radiation and medical oncology, then a common national data base should evolve. This minimum oncologic data base can then be used to generate paper forms on which initial information can be entered, either through key punching or mark sense reading and made available for terminal retrieval.

A second method is arranged so that the initial patient information on data base, problem list, plan, summary and progress notes are dictated onto forms in a fixed format which allows retrieval of certain key words and storage in the computer system. In the third, and probably optimum method, the minimum data base is combined with the initial required general medical base for oncologic patients and prepared for interactive terminal entry as described by SHULTZ *et al.* [6]. This system would allow the checking and correction of data while it is entered, the production of any necessary hard copy immediately and the selection of variables to be entered into a permanent retrievable file.

Some variation of this list of three methods will obviously be necessary for the inclusion of related centers and peripheral hospitals. It is completely possible to have a CRT-oriented input system at the major cancer center which works in conjunction with mark sense read paper forms in the peripheral related institutions. The minimal data base can be used by both systems and augmented by the complete data base which can be displayed on the CRT terminal. It is clear from our experience that the amount of information which can be collected on paper forms is limited to no more than 1,500 pieces of information and probably should not be more than 1,000. The information collectable on CRT screens by means of branching frame displays is almost unlimited. It now appears that the time is due for oncologists to get together and formulate a minimum oncologic data base. It is clear also that the modern cancer center can only operate effectively and lead to improved treatment and improved education if its data storage and recall systems are modernized. National study groups such as the Radiation Therapy Oncology Group and national organizations such as the American College of Radiology must be urged to begin the development of a common minimum oncologic data base. National granting agencies must be urged to support the rapid development of the necessary hardware and software for the complete computerization of oncologic data systems within the cancer centers.

References

1   FEINSTEIN, A. R.: Clinical judgment (Williams & Wilkins, Baltimore 1967).
2   HURST, J. W.: How to implement the Weed system. Arch. intern. Med. *128*:456-462 (1971).

3   HURST, J. W. and WALKER, H. K. (eds.): The problem oriented system (New York 1972).
4   OSLER, Sir W.: Aphorisms from his bedside teachings and writings (Schuman, New York 1950).
5   PHILLIPS, T. L.; DEFFEBACH, R. R.; CANTRIL, S. T.; CLAMPITT, S. M., and HARP, W.: Rapid access computerized data retrieval system for cancer patients (submitted to Radiology, 1972).
6   SCHULTZ, J. R.; CANTRILL, S. V., and MORGAN, K. G.: An initial operational problem oriented medical record system for storage, manipulation and retrieval of medical data; in HURST and WALKER. The problem oriented system, pp. 201-250 (Medcom Press, New York 1972).
7   WEED, L. L.: Medical records that guide and teach. New Engl. J. Med. *278*:593-599 652-657 (1968).
8   WEED, L. L.: Medical records, medical education and patient care. The problem oriented record as a basic tool (Case Western Reserve Univ. Press, Cleveland 1969).

Author's address: Dr. THEODORE L. PHILLIPS, Department of Radiology, University of California Medical Center, *San Francisco, CA 94122* (USA)

Front. Radiation Ther. Onc., vol. 8, p. 186
(Karger, Basel and University Park Press, Baltimore 1973)

Future Research Vistas

Gene De-repression and Clinical Cancer

J. H. FRENSTER

Abstract

Recent advances in the cell biology of human neoplastic diseases indicate the clinical importance of host defense mechanisms. These include specific activity by T and B lymphocytes, monocytes, macrophages, eosinophiles and fibroblasts directed against antigens on the surface of autochthonous neoplastic cells. These tumor-associated antigens are increasingly being recognized as the phenotypic expression of derepressed normal fetal genes. Such derepression of normal fetal genes is equally a feature of viral or chemical oncogenesis in animal neoplasms. Interestingly enough, gene derepression also is involved in the normal activation of immune lymphocytes and, thus, directed gene derepression may play an important rôle in the therapy as well as in the pathogenesis and diagnosis of neoplastic diseases. Gene derepression without gene alteration also raises the possibility of reversion from the neoplastic state to normal phenotypic gene expression within neoplastic cells. By means of a re-imposition of the normal repressed state for such oncolonic genes. [Nature New Biology *236*; 175–176 (1972)].

Author's address: JOHN H. FRENSTER, M. D., Assistant Professor of Medicine, Stanford Medical Center, *Stanford, CA 94305* (USA)

Front. Radiation Ther. Onc., vol. 8, pp. 187–192
(Karger, Basel and University Park Press, Baltimore 1973)

Discussions

PARSONS: A question for Dr. HELLMAN. You mentioned rotation of residents and staff throughout the organization. Do senior staff also rotate assignments?

HELLMAN: There is a director for each unit and he does not rotate. The junior attendants rotate assignments as well as the residents and trainees. There are 9 radiotherapists in the group, of whom 5 are senior and permanently assigned, 4 rotate.

PARSONS: Do you have an overall lay administrator? What do *you* do about administration?

HELLMAN: I have tried to avoid an administrative superstructure. I have an administrative associate. All the billing, collecting or purchasing are done through the individual hospitals, he acts only as a coordinator in this regard.

STEWART: As I understand the Boston situation, you are blessed with a sizeable number of hospitals within a reasonably short radius and I am impressed with what you say you have been able to do integrating this into a group. What do you think would be the limiting factors of distance if one were to attempt this organization over a larger geographic area?

HELLMAN: I don't know. That is a problem we have not had to face. I think it would be more of a problem but not insurmountable. I think the concept would work quite well. I think the right people are here to answer that question. Dr. JEROLD GREEN of the West Coast Cancer Foundation perhaps would comment. I understand there is considerable geographical separation between the components of the West Coast Cancer Foundation.

GREEN: I'd rather not at this point. Dr. ALAN SCHROEDER is going to talk in the afternoon session about integration of our Santa Rosa practice with our San Francisco practice. Santa Rosa is some 60 mi distant. In San Francisco there is an embryonic cancer advisory council. In Boston there has been a great recent development of radiation facilities not only in Harvard but also at Massachusetts General Hospital and Tufts and others.

I wonder what the community reaction is to supporting all these new projects simultaneously and what city-wide or community-wide organization is being carried out?

HELLMAN: I would like to correct you. Massachusetts General is part of Harvard but there are a number of different centers making major developments. As you know, FERNANDO BLOEDORN has a big center at Tufts, HERMAN SUIT at Massachusetts General. Our group has a large physical facility and people are saying 'Do we need all this, we could have too much in Boston?' It is very difficult to dissuade people from developing separate programs. In actual fact, FERNANDO BLOEDORN, HERMAN SUIT and I meet regularly. We have, in a way, separated the hospitals as to their primary orientation. This has been brought to a head by one hospital who tried to get active bidding between two of the three groups. It had a fixed opinion as to what it wanted, which did not conform with what we thought was rational. We went to the planning agency for assistance. They said 'You plan and then we will look and see if your plan is good.' The medical school stepped in, listened to what we said, agreed with us, and went to the hospitals and said 'This is the way it is going to be'. That is the way it was and it has worked. Our practical problems are obtaining new equipment. At this time, General Hospital, and I don't think I am misquoting this, is running a 2- to 3-week waiting period for patients and we are running a between 2- and 3-week waiting period. FERNANDO BLOEDORN is at capacity (I don't know if he has a waiting period). The people at B. U. are understaffed right now, but essentially all the major centers are running at capacity with waiting periods for initiation of treatment. It may appear as though we are oversupplied with equipment but there is good utilization. The commodity in short supply will always be skilled personnel, perhaps equipment, but certainly not patients. We are just being oversubscribed.

EINHORN: I would like to ask Dr. PHILLIPS if the problem-oriented data recall has been in function and how it is functioning? What difficulties did you find to date?

PHILLIPS: The complete problem-oriented record is in function in Vermont and I cannot really comment on that. Dr. BROWN is here from Vermont and might have some comments about that system. The one we have initiated in San Francisco, the paper-based system has been in function almost 1 year. About 2,500 cases have been entered. The major problem so far is getting consistency of input, eliminating unnecessary bits of information and in the future having the right kind of output manipulative programs to make the best use of the data. Without such an information system, not necessarily the system we have described, a cancer center cannot do its job properly. It cannot really know what it has done and change its approach rapidly enough to make the most rapid progress possible.

VAETH: Are there any other questions? Yes, Dr. BAKER?

BAKER: In the course of our discussions, much has been said about the importance of the rôle of research in cancer centers, I think we all agree on that, but I do suggest that there is a rôle for laboratory research in smaller academically oriented centers where clinical radiation oncology is being taught, not just the large medical school centers. I think the rôle of laboratory research in this context is one that has not really been mentioned this morning. Not only the residents, but the staff of these departments have to participate in research programs. The importance of the research program is the output. The output is not necessarily in new breakthroughs in cancer, but rather in the fact that it trains the residents and educates the staff man to think in a disciplined manner, to analyze problems and to develop imaginative methods. With this kind of environment and incentive, he takes the same questioning, imaginative attitudes back to the treatment of his patients, enabling him to treat his patient better.

PARSONS: I wish to direct a general question to all the speakers. Is it advisable to have all cancer patients in a hospital in one area or disperse them in general hospitals?

DE VITO: At the University of Washington, I think our physical plant as it stands makes it more desirable and more realistic to presume that the patients are not going to be segregated in a separate way nor even in a separate ward. We tend to admit patients to specific services which are ward-oriented because of nursing personnel and nursing habits. Philosophically, even at my young age, I am already beginning to feel old-fashioned. I am concerned that we have discarded the rotating internship and discarded the general clerkship so that students become specialized in the second year. They are becoming ultraspecialized in their own interests. They turn around 5 years later and say we have got to get together and understand what the others are doing. I would prefer not to see patients with malignancies separated physically and philosophically from the rest of the institution, if the institution is a training institution. So, with our population pattern and size in the State of Washington, particularly, I think I would prefer to see the patient in a general hospital facility.

VAETH: Perhaps Dr. EINHORN would comment on this. The Swedish system, as I understand it, is really going both ways.

EINHORN: The answer to Dr. PARSON's question is that I personally do not know which is better and nobody knows. But I feel that this solution is the one which gives us the best system of patient care. The patient is not afraid of an oncological center. The patient is afraid of having cancer whether he comes to the oncological center or not. If, as a physician, you do not want to tell your patient what kind of disease he has, of course, referring him to an oncological center is a bad thing because he will learn he has cancer. I believe that the patient always understands anyway and I believe this is more of a problem for the doctor than for the patient; the doctor, who is unable to discuss the situation with the patient and hides from the real problem. Once the patient knows what type of disease he has, he does not mind into which hospital he is admitted. I believe the primary diagnosis should be made in general departments, not specifically cancer departments, if possible. At that time no one is sure what kind of disease the patient has. We have been directing our attention to this problem you brought up. We have one psychiatrist and one psychologist on full time in our department to assist us. Our psychiatrist staff man confirms that once the patient knows what type of disease he has, he prefers to be in a department where everyone speaks freely about this disease and the doctors themselves are not afraid of cancer.

VAETH: Yes, Dr. RUBIN?

RUBIN: I think one of the things that is very important that has been surfaced by Dr. EINHORN's presentation is the fundamental issue we are facing in terms of training and practice. We have eluded to this in the conference in the introducing of the term 'radiation oncologist'. I mentioned in our teachers' meeting held at the West Coast Cancer Foundation at the University of the Pacific on Thursday that there are two papers being given back-to-back at the American Association for Cancer Education. One was on medical oncology, a new subspecialty. In medicine this is now recognized. The other was on radiation oncology, an 'emerging specialty'. It was the title of a paper my chief resident and I gave. What we addressed ourselves to was exactly how does one integrate programs in medical oncology and therapeutic radiology. Do we have two stems at some point in time, do they fuse together? But I think there is no question that a fusion of these two areas in the training period and the practice pattern are going to have to happen. JERZY EINHORN of Sweden has really taken that step and that commitment. That is an important thing for us to recognize in the United States. The integration of these two areas, of course, is practical and workable because it is under Dr. EINHORN's control. That is the way we would like it too, but I think that this is, leaving personalities aside, a very important commitment and a very important direction to recognize. All of us are going to have to recognize this concept in some form in each of our settings.

VAETH: Perhaps we can ask Dr. GOLDE what he feels about this. Is it unholy wedlock to think of medical oncologists and radiation oncologists under one roof? Sharing the same bed? Dr. GOLDE?

GOLDE: Well, we have it under one roof already at the University of California. Whether it could be the same individual or not, I am not absolutely certain. I believe that for practice in the United States we will still have a medical oncologist that is an internist who manages patients with neoplastic disease and a separate individual primarily using the radiotherapy modality. As I indicated in my talk, what we have tried to do is to bring these two people together on one ward. Our cancer ward contains patients that are being followed primarily by radiation therapy and patients that are being followed by the internist. We see each other each day on the ward and we make rounds on the same patients. It is the same nursing unit that looks after these patients. In the training period, which I believe to be the critical time for developing this cooperation, the trainees spend at least two months on each others' services. They get to know each other well and each acquires experience in the other's field of competence. It is doubtful that an internist could learn enough radiation therapy in these months so that he would sometime later be able to use this as a primary modality of care. Further, the cooperation developed at the training level must be supported later on, not based primarily on compatibility of individuals. We have taken steps to insure that there is a formalized cooperation by relating it to grant structure; if people are getting money from the same place, it makes cooperation somewhat easier. It also leaves room for arguments, but we think that when the individuals from both specialties are scheduled together, have their training programs integrated and where at least some of the funding is shared jointly, that the cooperative aspects are formalized and can be counted on though there may be changes in personnel.

VAETH: Dr. GOLDE it is interesting to hear you say that. My experience has been that anytime money comes into the scene, no matter at what level, cooperation tends to go out of the window. In the light of what Dr. GREEN mentioned and those of us who are in radiation therapy are aware, the so-called internship year can now be counted as a portion of the overall residency program. How should one shape the program for the radiation therapist trainee for that year of internship or first year of residency, specifically? Should he spend time in internal medicine? Should the trainee be working up patients with heart disease, etc., or should he be limiting his time strictly to medical oncology? And how much time?

GOLDE: That is a difficult question, one that we are just facing for the first time this year. I agree in a sense with Dr. DE VITO in that many of the trainees are specializing too early and I, too, regret the loss of the internship as a unit. I also feel that this very early subspecialization might carry with it certain risks in the future. In any case, I alluded to in my talk, the radiation therapy intern who has never had experience as a graduate physician; where should he get his first experience? We currently are giving a 6-months training on the medical oncology ward. We like to think that our medical oncology ward is a very strong internal medicine ward and that we do run it in the same way that the internal medicine wards are run in the university. On the other hand, it is clear that he is going to miss certain aspects of internal medicine that might be important to him later, particularly cardiology. So, in answer to your question, I think the minimum would be 6 months in medical oncology and in thinking about it, I do feel he should have additional experience on a general internal medicine ward.

VAETH: Dr. DE VITO, I feel that surgery is being neglected in this discussion. In the internship year, should the radiation therapy trainee have 6 months on the general surgical service? Should it be primarily surgical oncology or general surgery?

DE VITO: I am feeling older every minute because I believe a surgeon is first and foremost a technician. The man who is truly a surgeon must be able to perform the technical niceties that make him different from other physicians, that make him able to perform a service that other physicians cannot perform. To have meaningful surgical knowledge unfortunately requires prolonged experience and prolonged exposure to those things which make a technician. I don't think we should try to make trainees in all specialties of medicine part-surgeons. We would end up with failure. The important thing is for trainees, and this is at the medical student level, the resident level and the postgraduate level, to have an awareness of what is available in other specialties in medicine. This exposure can be generated for different specialties in different periods of time. Surgery is still a rather significant therapeutic modality in cancer and other areas. I feel very badly that medical students do not see what an operation is. I don't think that they have to learn to do an operation but they should see what they are asking their patients to undergo when they suggest that the patient see a surgeon. They should learn to appreciate the limitations of surgical therapy. They should spend time in the operating room, scrubbed or not scrubbed, but they should know what an operation is, the same as I should know what a patient is undergoing when he undergoes radiation therapy. I do not know how to give the therapy, I don't have to know how to calculate it, but I should be involved in seeing that patient when the patient is undergoing therapy. I guess I would like to see a rotating internship come back. It is interesting, Dr. VAETH, that the many good medical students who are interested in clinical medicine, when given the opportunity to elect senior-year courses, take a rotating internship in the senior year. The curriculum committees have structured it so that this is not what is designed. He is going to have a path, he is going to go straight, he is going to become very talented in his own narrow field. But the astute medical student, the better student and the honor student, elect the equivalent of a rotating internship because they know this need. Along this line I think we in education must realize that it is relatively rare to see a well qualified specialist fall on his face in managing a patient in his area of expertise. He does quite well. Where we see physicians fail is when they get on the fringe or just outside their area of superb competence. As educators, we must teach physicians who are required to get out on the edge of their area of competence to have some awareness of what they are doing and have some understanding of the potential pitfalls, so that they can ask for help and assistance.

VAETH: I tend to agree with you about the general rotating internship. I think that seeing this thing pass the American scene is bad news. But I know that this is certainly a source of argument. Dr. CANTRIL?

CANTRIL: I would like to comment. Dr. RUBIN has talked about chemotherapy and homeotherapy which is better know as medical oncology, as perhaps becoming integrated with radiotherapy. No one has mentioned that at least half, if not more, of the so-called chemotherapy, immunotherapy and hormonomanipulative therapy in this country is done by surgeons. This is a problem to which we have not addressed ourselves. Any surgeon can decide to do a surgical procedure and any physician, whether he is a general practitioner or medical oncologist, can prescribe drugs. We really are not addressing ourselves to this huge problem.

VAETH: Dr. EINHORN, will you comment on Dr. CANTRIL's remarks?

EINHORN: In Sweden and the other Scandinavian countries, any physician has the right to prescribe any drugs and he is doing it. Any surgeon can give chemotherapy and manipulative immunotherapy, but we try to have, in Sweden, some discipline in deferring areas of responsibility. We promote the position that expert consultation in oncology, medical or radiation, is readily available to the surgeons. If the surgeon wishes the non-surgical oncologist to treat the patient with chemotherapy, the patient is then referred to the medical oncology department. If the surgeon prefers to administer it, he is free to do that.